Sociology and Nursing

D0276322

Peter Morrall

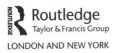

Routledge
Taylor & Francis Group

LONDON AND NEW YORK

First published 2001
by Routledge
11 New Fetter Lane, London EC4P 4EE

Simultaneously published in the USA and Canada
by Routledge
29 West 35th Street, New York, NY 10001

Reprinted 2002, 2004

Routledge is an imprint of the Taylor & Francis Group

Typeset in Times by Taylor & Francis Books Ltd
Printed and bound in Great Britain by Biddles Ltd,
King's Lynn, Norfolk

British Library Cataloguing in Publication Data
A catalogue record for this book is available from the British Library.

Library of Congress Cataloging in Publication Data
Morrall, Peter.
   Sociology and nursing / Peter Morrall.
   Includes bibliographical references and index.
   1. Nursing—Social aspects. 2. Social medicine.
   3. Medical sociology. I. Title. II. Series.
   [DNLM: 1. Sociology, Medical—Nurses' Instruction.
   2. Nursing Care. 3. Nursing. WA 31 M872s 2001]
   RT86.5 M66   2001
   610.73–dc21   00–042474

ISBN 0–415–20227–2 (hbk)
ISBN 0–415–20228–0 (pbk)

Contents

Introduction

Nursing practice without sociology is akin to sexual congress without orgasm – possible to enact, but highly unsatisfactory. It is the equivalent of entering a strange country without a map to explain the contours and pitfalls of the land. The traveller may eventually find the desired journey's end, but the route taken will be meandering and hazardous.

There is a dynamic and fundamental role for sociological knowledge within nursing (and health care generally). Sociology demystifies the nature of health and illness, highlights the social causes of disease and death, exposes power-factors and ethical dilemmas in the production of health care, and either directly or indirectly helps to create a discerning practitioner who then becomes capable of more focused and competent decision making.

However, I do not wish to overstate the case for sociology. The contribution of sociology must not be at the expense of the practical skills and instinctive 'caring', philosophy without which there is no discipline of nursing. Furthermore, the new millennium is an era of revolutionary ('hard') science and technology. Starting in the latter part of the twentieth century, unprecedented discoveries and 'reshaping' of human knowledge about the physical world have taken place. In the fields of physics, chemistry, mathematics, molecular biology, computing, pharmacology and medicine (both in terms of diagnosis and treatment), the accumulation of and transformation in knowledge have been nothing short of incredible. Through its foundations in critical thought, it is the task of sociology to examine just how authentic these changes are.

However, no matter how much hype there is surrounding the manufacture of theories to explain everything, and how effervescent are the promises for the detection of cures for all diseases, these developments in science and technology cannot (and should not) be categorised as mere fabrications. There has to be a fair and pragmatic balance between how much social science, biological science and pure 'nursing' is taught in the education of nurses. Moreover, the tendency for sociologists to lay to waste the factual and essential basis of every phenomenon is both unhelpful and ludicrous. Whilst sociology does provide legitimate, tangible and abundant insights into the organisation and shaping of matters relating to health and illness, much of what purports to be 'social science' is itself patently fatuous, obtuse, dogmatic and irrelevant to the everyday experiences of nurses (if not to everyone else).

We therefore have to be judicious in selecting what parts of the sociological enterprise are extracted and utilised in the critical examination of health and nursing. Not all knowledge is good knowledge, whether generated from the physical or the social sciences. Indeed, the underlying theme of this book is that a 'realistic' appraisal of what is health, and what can be expected of nurses, must be offered by sociologists. Moreover, sociology must be 'realistic' in what it can legitimately claim to be its contribution to human knowledge of the physical and the social world, including that of the domains of health and illness, and nursing.

Aims

Hence, the aims of this book are circumscribed and unpretentious. My intention is to provide the foundations for a sociological understanding of health issues, which can help nursing practitioners to manage the care of their patients more effectively – or at the very least more intelligently. Here sociology is presented as an 'applied' subject, substantiated by relevant theories and research. What I am not suggesting is that sociology should be an epistemological or pragmatic panacea, laying out well-defined pathways for politicians, policy makers, health service managers and clinical staff to follow. Whilst some elements of sociological knowledge can offer immediate and direct solutions to nursing issues, what is paramount is that the 'sociological imagination' is utilised to contextualise all nursing and health care action.

The specific objectives of the book are:

> To introduce sociological knowledge to nurses undertaking a wide range of undergraduate and postgraduate courses.

• To promote an inquisitive and reflective mode of conducting nursing work.

In order to achieve these goals fully, practitioners must both engage with the material offered here (including the further reading), and actively employ their sociologically inspired thinking into clinical practice. Even if only small transformations in the organisation and routines of the health system, and the reasoning and attitudes of nurses, are made as a result of reading this book, then it will mean that sociology has moved beyond its perennial status as an idealistic and mental-masturbatory '-ology'.

Format

Since the mid 1980s I have been teaching sociology to health-care workers at both undergraduate and postgraduate levels. Initially this was at the University of Teesside (formerly Teesside Polytechnic), and latterly at Leeds University. I have also taught modules and given lectures in health sociology in a number of other British as well as foreign universities. The range of students with whom I have shared the imagination of sociology over this time includes nurses from virtually all specialities (for example, general medicine and surgery; intensive care; paediatrics; learning disabilities; mental health; coronary care; accident and emergency; ear, nose and throat; district nursing; practice nursing; and community psychiatric nursing). Moreover, I have taught sociology to medical practitioners, midwives, health visitors, physiotherapists, occupational therapists, social workers, psychologists, audiologists and pharmacists, as well as to students from non-health-care disciplines such as sociology, social policy and criminology.

As a consequence of this experience I have selected, from an extensive list of possibilities, scholarship which has been cultivated most thoroughly within sociology (theoretically and/or empirically), and which students have indicated contributes most significantly to a better comprehension of the circumstances in which health care is enacted. Therefore, whilst I have included up-to-date sociological explanations and data, a substantial proportion of the material I have called upon is long-standing and seminal.

The structure and composition of the book forms, in educational terms, one learning 'module'. This includes an introduction and conclusion, and ten substantive topics. In each of the latter is the addition of a teaching and learning method which can be adopted for seminar discussions.

A collective effort, involving past students, colleagues at the University of Leeds and myself, sought to design a simple mechanism through which the principles of particular sociological perspectives could be demonstrated to have been understood, and could be explicitly shown to be applied to clinical practice. The mechanism we assembled is what I have called the Practice Grid (Appendix 1). The way it works is very straightforward, but has proven to be remarkably functional. After each lecture students are invited to complete the three columns in the Practice Grid diagram. The first column refers to the theory to be applied, the second to the principles that can be extrapolated from that theory, and the third to the specific implications for the area of practice in which the student works. It is probably of most benefit for the student to have digested the content of the lecture and the suggested further reading before the exercise is tackled. The completed grid can then be used to generate discussion in tutorials and seminars, as a type of formative assessment, in the preparation of summative assignments, and to supplement nursing and organisation planning in hospitals and the community.

Content

The chapters are organised in a logical, unfolding and maturing configuration. That is, there is an overall rationale of moving the student from the discipline's 'tools of the trade' (i.e. the main sociological perspectives), through to bedrock concepts underpinning nursing work (i.e. health, science and power), and on to particular sociological concerns pertinent to health and nursing. However, although the input in each chapter has been arranged under particular topics, this has created arbitrary and erroneous divisions. That is, the substance of each chapter is interlinked with that of all of the chapters.

The starting point for a rigorous appreciation of any academic subject must be its principals. The chemist has to learn the rules of experimentation, the physicist laws of mass and motion, the mathematician geometrical formulae and the physiologist the functions of molecules and organs. Once commanded and internalised, these principals can be drawn upon to make sense out of physical or social events. However, such learning is never easy. Preconceived beliefs are challenged, and new ideas and alternative ways of viewing the world have to be grappled with. This is not an option.

An initiate of sociology must contend with the conjecture and concepts associated with the discipline. Once comprehended, the essence of sociology can be utilised to help shed light on how the social context influences health and illness, and nursing practice. Consequently, Chapter 1 contains an overview of the main theoretical traditions of sociology. These theories, in one form or another, are used as perceptual scalpels in the subsequent chapters. A reading and grasp of this chapter is paramount to an appreciation of the rest of the content of the book, and should be referred back to during the reader's excursion through each of the subsequent chapters. Although additional conceptual considerations will be presented at other points in the book, these all have their roots in the founding theories established in Chapter 1.

Chapter 2 deals with definitions of health, illness and disease. Here, it is demonstrated that the meaning of health-related terms is extremely difficult to establish in any concrete and unambiguous way. That is, despite 'health' and 'ill-health' being the primary focus of nursing, what these states signify is not at all fixed, either with respect to the practitioner's interpretation of them, or how they are experienced by the patient.

Science (primarily the 'hard' variety) has traditionally formed the foundation of what Western society at large and also the profession of medicine (and to a lesser extent the discipline of nursing) hold as convincing knowledge. Chapter 3 starts with an account of the history of scientific ideas. Contemporary contention over the efficacy and accuracy of scientific scholarship (including that of bio-medicine and nursing) are then reviewed.

In Chapter 4 the theme of power in health care is discussed. The ways in which doctors and nurses perform a social role in the control of so-called 'deviant' behaviour (i.e. 'illness') is evaluated. There is also an examination of how power enters into the consultation process between health-care practitioners and patients, and how the move towards reconstituting the status of the citizen, and the creation of an empowered health 'consumer', has affected the practitioner–patient relationship.

The historical and present status of the professional is then examined in Chapter 5. The background to the procurement of a professional identity by medicine, and the desire for such social prestige by nursing, are evaluated. The influence of medical practitioners in a modern and disputatious health system is then compared to that of nurses.

The analysis of professional power and status leads to an explication in Chapter 6 of the effect of the medical profession and health industry on people's lives. Here there is an assessment of the positive and/or negative results of the intrusion of medical and health ideologies into all aspects of human existence.

In Britain, and probably most other societies, whether in the West or developing world, an individual's position in the social stratum will have a much more significant impact on her or his health than, for example, genetic predisposition, or exposure to pathogenic micro-organisms. That is, long-term unemployment, poverty and living in overcrowded and polluted environmental conditions, signify highly in the aetiology of serious illness and early death. This crucial sociological observation of the social causes of disease and death is the focus of Chapter 7.

The next three chapters are about what have been, and what still may be, taboo issues. Chapter 8 is about sex. Sex is a misunderstood and greatly misrepresented human faculty both in society at large and most certainly in the health-care setting. Today, with doctors and nurses acknowledging the 'holistic' needs of their patients, the immense suffering caused through sexually transmitted diseases, and the social consequences of inadequate health education aimed at preventing unwanted pregnancy, there can no excuse for not addressing sex head-on.

Mental disorder is one of the most common but also most controversial conditions dealt with by the health service. Is it in fact an illness? Alternatively, is it a 'manufactured' category used to contain (for example, through the use of medication and enforced hospitalisation) disruptive elements in society? If it is so common, why do people suffering from it continue to be so stigmatised? In Chapter 9 the history of the treatment of mad people is described, and competing explanations from various professional and academic groups are explored.

The last of the ten substantive issues covered in the book is, aptly, death. Specifically, the social context of the end of human life, and the reaction of health-care practitioners to dying and death, are the topics for Chapter 10. Death, like sex and madness, is an unavoidable fact of human existence. Why then, especially in Western countries, is it so hidden from view, and either not talked about at all or couched in euphemism? A number of classical sociological studies, describing how doctors and nurses 'shape' the dying process to fit both their own projections of 'a good death' and the requirements of their organisation, are outlined.

The conclusion of the book contains a commentary about the main themes that emerge from the material covered. Here I also call into question the traditional distrust of health-care conceptions and practices by sociologists, and suggest that there must be a limit to purely sceptical sociological analysis. The sociological imagination applied to health care should be ambitious in the exposing of myths, inequalities and the abuse of power. But, as with climax during sexual congress, the successful culmination of sociological activity in health care is best attained when participants collaborate. The pilgrimage toward a demythologised and equitable health system needs not just one epistemological blueprint, but all that are available.

Chapter 1

Imagination

> to understand the changes of many personal milieux we are re-
> quired to look beyond them. ... To be able to do that is to possess
> the sociological imagination.
>
> (Mills 1959: 10/11)

Sociologists imagine the world differently compared with the way it
is viewed for example, by psychologists, and biologists, or by those
who proffer 'common sense'. In this chapter 'the sociological
imagination' is delineated through an exploration of three major
theoretical frameworks. I am using the term 'theoretical framework'
to describe the grouping of perspectives which may have subtle
differences that distinguish them, but which have similar philosophical routes, and complementary observations to make about the
organisation of society and human action.

The first theoretical framework I have chosen regards society as
both existing and having a set of configurations that to a greater or
lesser extent induces humans to behave and think in preordained
ways, including that of 'being sick'. As an alternative to this
structural understanding of human behaviour and thinking, which
can be interpreted as viewing all thought and behaviour as
'determined' by society, the second explanatory genre projects the
notion of individual volition. That is, it is argued that humans can
and do direct their own lives. The third theoretical framework has
gained popularity in nursing literature in the last couple of decades,
and has been extracted from a range of sociological theorising that
aims to 'deconstruct' reality (including the actuality of 'disease') in
one way or another.

As with all academic subjects, certain people have made major
contributions to sociology throughout its relatively short history.

This chapter will concentrate on a small number of the 'founders' of sociology and their respective perspectives.

There is nothing totally 'natural', 'God-given' or inevitable about personal and social behaviour. Falling in love, committing a crime, achieving success in a career, or being ill, are all influenced by social factors. The basis of the 'sociological imagination' is to look beyond the obvious, and to challenge both our own preconceived ideas and those of others. This is of particular importance when those with power in society hold prejudicial views about already vulnerable and dispossessed people. Above, all, it is to always ask the question 'why', and to keep on asking the question 'why'!

It was C. Wright Mills (1959) who pointed to the connection between 'private troubles' and 'public issues'. Whatever we undergo as individuals (and this applies to emotions, pain, disease and cognition) our social surroundings have either helped create, or are affected by, these experiences. For example, the private trouble of losing a loved one in a car accident is a public issue in that both the amount of money governments put into road safety, and the degree to which a society values commodities such as cars, are linked to the number of people who are killed on the roads. The private trouble of being diagnosed as having cancer is also a public issue as either directly or indirectly it relates to health policy and health-service resources, which in turn are connected with social values. Better health promotion strategies installed by government and health agencies, a greater political will at local and national levels to improve the physical environment, more money ploughed into cancer research and treatment rather than, for example, arms technology, may have prevented that person's malignant tumour. The private issue of depression is a public issue in the sense that this 'internal' condition may have been precipitated by alienating and dehumanising social circumstances.

Social events and social relationships are not taken at face value by the sociologist. Conventional wisdom is tested to see whether or not it stands up to the scrutiny of research and well-worked-out theorising. Many prevailing ideas do not. For example, it was 'common sense' for white imperialists and colonialists from Europe to believe that black Africans were sub-human. Another 'common-sense' judgement was made by the ruling elite in the Victorian age that the mad should be locked up in asylums, the poor put in workhouses and criminals transported to Australia. Not so long ago, it was 'common sense' to regard women as not only the 'weaker sex' physically but also intellectually.

Everyone, unless extremely young or lacking cognitive ability through, for example, intoxication or dementia, in some way studies their social world. The veritable 'man on the Clapham omnibus' may ponder over why there is such conspicuous opulence (in the form of what is displayed in shop windows, personal adornment, and material possessions such as cars) alongside scores of young people begging on the streets. He may speculate about the patent differences between one residential area of the city and another with respect to the ethnic make-up of its population, the condition of housing and the physical ambience.

The formal study of society, however, was initiated by Auguste Comte (1798–1857) who in 1838 conceived of the term 'sociology', and thereby inaugurated a new academic discipline. Many of Comte's ideas are to found in the work of later theorists. The literal interpretation of the word 'sociology', coming from the Latin 'socius' and 'ology' is the study of companionship. My own definition is as follows: 'Sociology is the rigorous investigation of social phenomena using systematic theorising and methodical research procedures.' It is the use of theories and research (which have been scrutinised through exacting peer review and debate) that separates 'common sense' from substantive knowledge.

Of course, the 'man on the Clapham omnibus' may, through his own reasoning or a lucky guess, have reached the same conclusions as social theorists and researchers after perhaps years of theorising and data collection. But he will not, except through assertion and belligerence, be able to sustain his point of view, whereas the evidence of the sociologist could be substantial enough to warrant serious attention and response.

However, there is much controversy over what sociology actually is as subject, and about the role of theory and research in the analysis of society. It is exceptional to find two sociologists who agree with each other about all aspects of the sociological enterprise. Internal disagreement can be seen as 'productive' in that organised deliberation (for example, at conferences and in academic journals) can tease out inconsistencies and defects in a theoretical concept or in the procedures and results of a research project. On the other hand, the perpetual arguments and disparate propositions disgorged by sociologists may demonstrate the fallibility of the subject.

In the 1960s and 1970s in Britain and other Western countries, sociology became established as an academic subject in universities and schools. However, in the 1980s, under the Tory government in Britain, sociology was denigrated as a worthless subject and also judged as too left wing politically for a radical 'new-right' administration to stomach, to the point whereby, infamously, Margaret Thatcher announced that 'there was no such thing as society' – indicating, therefore, that there was nothing for sociologists to study. Given the subject's lamentable record in predicting social events, and its undoubted Marxist bias at the time, both of these accusations had some justification.

Whilst never suffering from a reduction in the amount of students who wished to study the subject at secondary or tertiary levels, its low standing in the eyes of the general public was exemplified in a notorious television advertisement for British Telecommunications during the 1980s. The scene is of a caring if anxious mother talking with her son on the telephone about his school examination results. Miserably, he explains to his mother that he has failed everything except sociology, and this he patently considers to be of little compensation. His mother, enacting the vocal intonation and gestures of a stereotypical Jewish mother, counters with the (for sociologists) cringe-making phrase 'well, at least it's an "ology" '.

Moreover, the intellectually corrupt condition of sociology was epitomised with publication in 1975 of the novel *The History Man* by Malcolm Bradbury, an academic himself at a red-brick university in England. Despite its rather misleading title, this otherwise well-written and perspicacious book (which was also produced as a television drama), told the story of a sexually exploitative and anti-establishment lecturer, whose superlative aggrandisement of sociological prognostications served to signify the over-ambitious presumptions of the discipline. That is, the central character of the book, Howard Kirk, was a ridiculous figure who represented an epistemology that had overreached itself, and in doing so appeared as absurd as Kirk himself.

In the 2000s, however, sociology, whilst not chastened in its aspirations and notwithstanding colossal amounts of self-indulgent and impotent theorising over the previous twenty years, has been revitalised. For example, the eminent professor of sociology and Director of the London School of Economics, Anthony Giddens, has had much influence on the thinking of the British 'New Labour' government elected in 1997, with his theorising on social democratic programmes under the epithet of the 'Third Way' (Giddens 1998). Giddens also delivered the prestigious BBC 'Reith' Lectures in 1999, which attract worldwide audiences and participation by other senior academics and political commentators.

The work of the American sociologist Amitai Etzioni on 'communitarianism' (1998), and that of the German social theorist Ulrich Beck on 'risk society' (1992) have also been influential in Western politics. These commentators, in different ways, have pointed to the consequences of immense social change and the need for communities and social systems to adjust in order to reduce the damage to society and its inhabitants from these changes.

Moreover, Ian Christie has argued that while the pronouncements of sociologists may still not be at the forefront of the public's consciousness, issues affecting the lives of individuals and communities (for example, crime, the disintegration of traditional family life, poverty, unemployment, stress at work, patterns of disease) are defined in terms of their social causes and consequences, and social solutions are sought (Christie 1999). Classical sociological research techniques (i.e. the survey and interviewing) are routinely employed to assess crime rates, explore family dynamics, analyse voting habits and in assessing the health needs of communities and individuals.

Nursing has incorporated social factors into most if not all of its educational programmes. Whether it be the study of childbirth, breast cancer, coronary vascular disease or schizophrenia, the inclusion of social factors in the aetiology, care and treatment of patients and their families are *de rigueur*. Medicine, whilst far more resistant to the 'contamination' of its natural scientific foundation, has accepted sociology in its undergraduate training for decades. Furthermore, apart from the obvious case of psychiatric medicine, heavily influenced by Sigmund Freud's sociological account of the effects of culture and the family on the unconscious psychological mechanisms of the individual (Bocock 1976), postgraduate medical education specialising purely in social science applied to disease is now not unusual. For example, the University of Leeds offers surgeons a course in the psycho-social aspects of oncology.

Structure

The structural paradigm in sociology posits that humans belong to social groups and that it is membership of these groups that to a greater or lesser degree dictates behaviour. Specifically, the institutions of society (for example, the health system; the police service; the law courts; the educational system; the family; business and commerce; the media) and the ways in which society is divided (on the basis of, for example, social class; gender; ethnicity; age; and geographical region) set out the boundaries for human performance. Structuralist theorising has infiltrated many areas of health policy.

For Comte (1853), there were general laws of social structure and development, just as the chemist or physicist was able to state that laws existed in the physical world and thereby shaped that world. He perceived society as analogous to human anatomy and physiology. Each structure of society like the structures of the human body (for example, the heart, liver, brain and colon) was interconnected. Each was dependent on the other parts, and this was to become more so as society progressed through its historical stages towards greater complexity.

Hence, Comte was holistic in his approach to comprehending society. He saw society as being made up of interrelating parts, but also as a 'whole' entity. If we look at the human body we know that it is made up of billions of molecules but we can't hope to appreciate fully what it is to be a 'human' by merely examining one minute constituent element of the body. Of course, mapping out the structure, composition and purpose of each gene may be incredibly useful in the search for causes of. disease and certain personality traits, but on its own it will not provide a comprehensive grasp of human spirituality, motivation, personality, athleticism, sexuality, love or thinking. Similarly, for Comte, it is society as a whole and society's institutions and large-scale structures that have to be analysed rather than the activities of individuals.

Like Comte, and being greatly influenced by him, Emile Durkheim (1858–1917) contributed much to the development of sociology as an academic subject and in particular to the formulation of the *functionalist* perspective. *Functionalism* attempts to explain why society is the way it is by portraying all of its institutions (for example, those associated with the law, education or health) as having a purpose. For Durkheim, as for Comte, society is more than the sum of its parts. That is, society has an existence of its own which is not just the aggregate of behaviour exhibited by its members, and cannot be comprehended by the examination of such individual behaviour. Sociological research should seek out social facts, and use methods (specifically, the social survey) that attest to the structural impositions of society on human behaviour.

Hence, Durkheim contested the reductionist idea that social acts (for example, marriage, attending school, being ill, inner-city riots or working as a nurse) could be explained by reference to the behaviour and motivation of individuals. For example, Durkheim (1966; orig. 1897) argued that the rate of suicide is more to do with how society is ordered than to do with the individual's personality or state of (mental) health. Ostensibly the most personal of all acts, killing oneself, was induced or frustrated by such 'social facts' as the structure of family ties.

Durkheim regarded the various social structures and institutions as operating cohesively for society. If conflict occurs (as for example between trade unions and employers) then eventually 'adaptation' will ensue (deals will be made or one side will win) and therefore social stability is maintained. In this way societies develop evolutionarily rather than through revolution. Even the class structure is accepted as functional to the successful working of society.

Social order for the functionalist is maintained through the process of socialisation. Families, schools and other socialising institutions inculcate members of a particular society with 'acceptable' values. Those who go against the consensus of opinion and challenge the dominant system of ideas are treated by society as 'deviants'.

However, the functionality of social institutions is questionable. Take the example of the family. For the functionalist Ronald Fletcher (1962), industrialisation required a smaller family which was geographically mobile. The 'nuclear family' of the industrial age, composed of two heterosexual (married) adults and a limited number of children, served capitalist society well. Its reduced membership and weaker family ties, compared to that of the much larger 'extended' variety of agrarian economies and early capitalist development, meant that it could move to where work could be found (i.e. wherever business decided to create new jobs). Moreover, this family arrangement gave succour to its members. Children could be socialised, sexual energy contained, and domestic and employment tasks allocated on the basis of gender.

However, social relationships have altered irrevocably, and the claim of functionality for the family is somewhat ambiguous. The family in Western countries in the third millennium is structurally very different to that considered by Fletcher. In Britain, less than a quarter of households fit the nuclear family stereotype of a married (or cohabiting) couple living with their own children. Marriage itself is being entered into much later, and 40 per cent of those who marry will divorce – the highest rate amongst countries of the European Union (Macionis and Plummer 1998). In England and Wales, 38 per cent of births are outside marriage – again the highest rate in the European Union (Office for National Statistics (ONS) 1999). As a social ritual, however, marriage remains popular. Nine out of ten people still do get married at some point in their lives (Hardyment 1998).

One-person households make up over 25 per cent of all households, and approximately one-third of children are born to unmarried parents – the vast majority of whom (80 per cent) have formed stable relationships (Macionis and Plummer 1998). But couples who have children after they marry are more likely to stay together (as measured after five years) than those who cohabit and have children (ONS 1999). The vast majority of women are now in paid employment, although the greatest growth in female labour has been in the service sector, and is either temporary or part time (Allan 1999).

Most people have sex before marriage, and the advent of effective contraception has given women more control over their sexuality and reproduction. Moreover, changes in attitude towards sex and marriage, and the 25 per cent increase in life expectancy that occurred in the twentieth century, have led to the appearance of novel forms of social alliances. Specifically, the 'restructured step-family' has been created. Individuals may enter into a series of monogamous relationships during their lifetime, and bring with them children from previous relationships.

Much more provocative to conceptions of 'normal' family life, however, is the presence and growing acceptability of gay family units, which may even include adopted children. In 1999 the House of Lords ruled that a homosexual couple, where there was evidence of long-term interdependence in one household, for the purposes of the law, could be defined as a family.

Changes in the ways in which humans form close ties does not necessarily, however, undermine the functionalist project. Whilst it has become normal for right-wing politicians to regard anything other than the 'traditional family' to be the cause of every social problem (for example, crime, truancy and unemployment) it could be argued that these new arrangements may still be functional for both the individuals and society at large. It may be that in post-industrial society different arrangements are necessary.

On the other hand, the break-up of the family may be extremely and patently dysfunctional for some sections of society. For example, the increase in single-occupancy households seems to have more benefits for women than men. A study by Richard Scase (1999) for the Economic and Social Research Council (ESRC) concluded that the single-person household will predominate by 2010, and that the lifestyles of single women are much more fulfilling and healthy compared to the 'sad culture' of single men. Men living alone are less likely than women to have visits from friends, to cook for themselves or have meals with others, visit the theatre or cinema, or to partake in spiritual and self-awareness activities, or to take regular exercise. Characteristically, men go to the pub, eat take-away food and watch videos. Women are much more self-confident in the single lifestyle, and are inclined to engage in longer-term sexual and emotional relationships, whereas the social isolation of men may be linked to the huge rise in male suicide.

Functionalism attempts to explain social activities (such as marriage) in terms of the consequences of these activities, and this is a major criticism of the perspective. For example, the functionalist commenting on the health system of a nation may say that it exists (and has taken the shape that it has) because it satisfies the needs of that society. Consequently, if asked the question 'how are the health needs of this society satisfied', the functionalist's reply would be something like 'its health needs are met through its health system'. If asked the question 'why are most nurses women', a functionalists rejoinder might be 'women are most suited to nursing work'. Therefore, only circular (or 'teleological') answers are forthcoming. There is little appreciation of other factors that need to be considered in these two examples, such as how the heath of poor people does not seem to be attended to adequately by the health system, and that men could (and do) discharge the duties of a nurse.

Moreover, structural feminists have argued that society is based on patriarchy (Millett 1977). That is, notwithstanding advances made by women in the political sphere and the workplace, men overall are still dominant. The top jobs in industry, education and science, are occupied by men, and masculine values (for example, competitiveness and aggression) continue to be pre-eminent in society. Therefore, the demarcation of society by gender may be more functional for men than for women. The reason that nursing is carried out mainly by women is, as with housework and other menial work in society, the consequence of a structural exclusion of women from positions of power and prestige.

As with structural feminism, the structuralism of Karl Marx (1818–1883), however, offers insights that supplant basic functionalist explanations (although there is still an element of teleology within Marxist theorising). Marx's theories and his concepts, most of which are connected to his unique account of history (emphasising the importance of the economy in shaping our behaviour and destiny), relate to his observations of the capitalist system as it was in the nineteenth century. However, whilst his overall thesis on social evolution has been discredited, his reasoning about the intricacies and corrupting effects of industrialisation remains of importance in the twenty-first century.

For example, in his earlier work Marx (1959; orig. 1844) argued in his publications that the way capitalist society was structured resulted in people becoming 'alienated' from their own humanity. He believed that 'work' was an essential human requirement because it allowed individuals to express their creativity, and enabled social co-operation to take place between people. Capitalism, for Marx, encouraged working practices that meant restricted or removed creativity, and replaced social co-operation with interpersonal exploitation. As 'employees' in capitalist enterprises, people were no longer in control of what they were doing, became estranged from the completed product, and gained little satisfaction from their work. Work becomes under capitalism something one does for others for money. In Marxist terms, people have become 'wage labourers' or even 'wage slaves'.

In the twenty-first century, there is likely to be a huge growth in the number of computer operatives who sit in large office 'warehouses' answering telephone calls concerning insurance, banking and telecommunication services. Nearly a million people are employed in conditions that engender little job satisfaction, and produce a high turnover of staff and strikes (Wazir 1999). The work of these computer operatives in these warehouses corresponds to that of the nineteenth-century 'sweat-shops' and twentieth-century assembly lines.

Marx in his later work (1971; orig. 1867) was to highlight the connection between the economic 'base' of a society and its 'superstructure'. The economic base is made up of two sets of people. These are, on the one hand, the people who do the work, and on the other, those who force them to do so, or employ them. According to Marx, throughout history these two groups have been in tension with one another. In ancient society it was slave against slave-owner, in medieval times it was feudal Lord against serf, and in the industrial age the proletariat (i.e. the working class) against the bourgeoisie (the middle class). The economic base is also made up of the machinery and technology used in the production of goods and services. The superstructure of a society is all the other institutions and their concomitant patterns of belief (for example: religion; the family; health systems; education; criminal justice; politics; and the media).

Marx believed that it was the conflict between the 'exploited' and the 'exploiters' in each type of economic system that led to change. He anticipated that capitalist countries would eventually move towards a system without social inequality (i.e. communism).

Exploitation occurs for Marx at various levels under capitalism. One level is in the workplace where people work in dangerous or filthy surroundings with monotonous jobs and have little say in the running of the factory or business. At a more structural level of analysis Marx recognised that workers generated wealth but only ever received part of it. The rest, which Marx called 'surplus value' went to the bosses (i.e. the capitalists who owned the factory or business).

The implication is that the economic base actually directs the shape of everything else in society. For Marx, the capitalist form of economy is supported by an ideology which favours the interests of the ruling class, foments a fetish for owning commodities, and 'mystifies' the reality of high levels of exploitation. The ruling class disseminates this ideology via for example, the media and the education system.

Marx's conception of social class, based on a division between those who own the 'means of production' (i.e. factories, property) and capital and those who do not, can also be applied to the relationship between countries across the globe. That is, the world can be seen to be split into two distinct socio-economic areas. The 'first' or 'developed world', consisting of Western Europe, North America, Japan, and Australasia, had been at the forefront of industrialisation. Sheer exploitation, through colonisation and beneficial trade arrangements, resulted in the first world becoming extremely wealthy compared with the 'third' or 'developing' world.

There is, in between the first and third worlds, the second world, made up of an inconstant list of countries, depending on levels of economy production. This list has included at one time or another, the former Union of Socialist Soviet Republics, Brazil, Mexico and the 'tiger economies' of Singapore, Taiwan, South Korea, Thailand and Malaysia. The economies of these countries were regarded as 'transitional'. That is, they were on the way to full industrialisation, but did not have the economic clout of those in the first world. However, it is not always clear whether or not some of these countries are heading for the economic high ground or are slipping back into financial disorder, and therefore falling further down the world's hierarchy of industrial nations.

China is of course in the ascendancy industrially, and has the potential to become not only a military and economic superpower alongside the United States of America (USA), but to form another major 'trading block' to rival those of North America and the European Union. In 1999, China signed a trade agreement with the USA liberalising its commercial practices, and joined the World Trade Organisation, thereby formally entering the capitalist market economy, allowing external businesses access to its 1.2 billion consumers.

Rather than, as envisaged by Marx, a collapse of capitalism, there has been a globalisation of Western ideas about how economies should be run. Capitalism is virtually pandemic; businesses cut across national boundaries; and Western-orientated financial organisations such as the World Bank and the International Monetary Fund are, at times, instructing directly third-world and second-world governments on fiscal management.

However, the World Trade Organisation, whose agenda on global investment and trading procedures is dominated by the large industrial countries, came under intense pressure in 1999 from anti-capitalist and environmental protesters to change its policies to allow poorer countries more favourable terms. Serious street riots occurred in the USA city of Seattle where negotiating teams from 135 countries had met to discuss trade agreements.

But, the economic strength of the industrialised nations has had another effect on the rest of the world – that of 'cultural imperialism'. By 'cultural imperialism' I am referring to exporting of Western values concerning, for example, material possessions, mass entertainment and health, to societies where people have traditionally had very different ways of existing. Moreover, technological advances in communication systems, particularly that of the Internet, increase the rate and depth of Western practices into other cultures.

Moreover, there has not only been a globalisation of Western culture, but also of Western inequalities. Wealth is not shared equally between the developed and the under-developed world, or within developed-world countries, and this pattern is replicated with the asymmetric distribution of technology – the 'digital divide'. Of course, just as televisions, videos and American-branded soft drinks can be found in the most impoverished of communities, it is likely (if it is in the interests of business) that in future years we will see personal computers in the most underprivileged areas. The selling of computers to those who have little money even for the basics of everyday existence is no different to the pharmaceutical, tobacco, chemical and baby-food industries marketing products in the third world which have either been banned in the West or are considered to be too risky to use. Capitalism as an economic structure has no inherent ethical dynamic.

Interaction

Max Weber (1864–1920) has made a considerable contribution to sociology, and his work retains its influence. His work gave birth to a multitude of social-science theories with a wide range of application (for example, symbolic interactionism; ethnomethodology; phenomenology). The underlying philosophies of many other theories also have their origins in his work (for example, constructionism and post-modernist theorising). Moreover, there is synchronicity between Weber's theoretical stance and the core tenets of holistic nursing care, a large proportion of nursing research and elements of health promotion programmes.

Weber's ideas can be regarded as a direct challenge to the structuralism of both Durkheim and Marx. According to Weber, society had to be analysed at the level of the individual rather than at the level of social structure. Sociologists should, therefore, be concerned with investigating the 'meaning' behaviour has for the individual. However, humans are not merely unitary organisms operating in a social vacuum. Unlike the reductionism of the psychologist or biologist, who address human behaviour through the narrow perspective of mental functioning and physiology, Weber perceived humans as 'social actors'. That is, what humans do and think is inexorably connected to the social setting in which they live out their daily lives, and to the broader society to which they belong. For example, the meaning individuals give to their social relationships will be different (i.e. more impersonal, isolating and instrumental) in a society where communications via the Internet replace face-to-face interaction (Nie and Erbring 2000).

Hence, human behaviour is not just the action of isolated individuals, but is 'social action'. However, and this is the crucial difference between structuralism and Weber's social action theory, the meaning individuals give to their action is what creates society. Society, is not, as Durkheim would have it, 'greater than the sum of its parts', but is only 'the sum of its parts'. That is, people react to their environment, and offer interpretations of social events. Therefore, people consciously make and alter the social order around them, rather than, as the structuralists propose, having society impinging on human free will. Weber's concentration on the individual meant that he disagreed with Durkheim's idea that universal laws of social behaviour could be discovered.

Consequently, Weber rejected 'objective' sociological methods of research. He argued for an 'interpretative' method through which the sociologist would intuitively or empathetically come to understand human behaviour and therefore the working of society. The German word 'verstehen' is used to describe this thorough comprehension of the meaning social actors give to their behaviour. Participant observation is the Weberian research method of choice. Here the researcher enters the world of the people she or he is studying, as it is argued that it is only possible to appreciate in-depth what is happening in any given social situation if you become part of it.

Against Marx's notion of historical change, Weber argued, for example, that it was the Protestant Reformation that stimulated the growth of the capitalist mode of production. Specifically, it was the Protestant Calvinists who were responsible for encouraging value to be given to working hard and individual achievement. The Calvinists believed that if their endeavour was successful then this indicated that they would be chosen to enter heaven on death. The wealth they accrued was not spent on 'conspicuous consumption', but reinvested in business and commerce. This had the effect, reasoned Weber, of building up the industrial economies of the West. Therefore, Weber contradicted Marx by pointing to elements of the superstructure (i.e. religious belief) of society as being the catalyst for change rather than the economic base.

Again, Weber disagreed with Marx over who had power in society. Marx saw power in the hands of the dominant economic group (i.e. a ruling class who owned the means of production). But Weber believed that people other than those with economic supremacy could hold power in society. Weber's point was that certain 'status groups' may have more esteem and influence than those who own business enterprises or even large amounts of wealth.

For example, in liberal democracies, an individual born into the bottom of the social hierarchy may rise to the top through gaining educational and professional qualifications. The daughter of a bus driver may attain the high social status of lawyer if she is successful at school and university. The winners of the national lottery might not automatically enter into the elite stratum of society if they are regarded as belonging to the 'wrong class'. However, the children of 'new money' might achieve high social status if put on the track of private education, by their parents, or if a career in a reputable line of business is 'bought' for them.

Moreover, collections of people can thrive in the social hierarchy by campaigning successfully for increased control over their work and greater remuneration (both financial and in terms of employment 'perks'). This has been the history of the medical and legal professions, and is the direction sought by the leaders of nursing, physiotherapy, occupational therapy, counselling and clinical psychology. The technique used by such groups, argued Weber, is that of 'social closure'. In order to advance the status of a group, its members make it increasingly difficult to belong to that group by elevating the requirements for entry, and making the claim that only its members have the authority and expertise to operate in a well-defined area of work.

Weber's notion of social status is consistent with the method used by policy makers to categorise the population into occupational groups. Throughout the twentieth century the Registrar General placed individuals within a hierarchy of occupations, which then enabled researchers and governments to assess trends in, for example, employment, crime, residence and health (see Table 1.1). The Registrar General's schema contained five categories, ranging from professional to unskilled occupations.

Table 1.1   Registrar General's classification of occupations

Category	Occupation type	Examples
I	Senior professions	Doctors, lawyers, university lecturers
II	Intermediate professions	Teachers, nurses, managers
III (non-manual)	Skilled workers	Clerks, cashiers
III (manual)	Skilled workers	Coal miners, bricklayers, electricians
IV	Semi-skilled	Bus conductors, postmen/postwomen
V	Unskilled	Labourers, porters, refuse collectors

Source: OPCS (1991)

The use of a standard measure of occupational status also allowed for statistics to be compared from one period to another, or one geographical area to another. However, this system came under increasing criticism for excluding the very rich (who may not be 'employed' as such and therefore could not be classified by a formal occupational title), most women (by-and-large they were classified by the occupation of their husband), and the unemployed. Moreover, the status of some jobs had changed considerably over the years; many occupations had disappeared with the dissolution of heavy manufacturing industries; and new types of employment had been created due to technological developments. Consequently, the Economic and Social Research Council (ESRC) has proposed adjustments to the Registrar General's system, and introduced eight rather than five categories (see Table 1.2).

Table 1.2   Revised social classification (ESRC)

Category	Occupation
1	Doctors, lawyers, scientists Employers and managers (larger organisations)
2	Nurses, teachers Employers and managers (smaller organisations)
3	Secretaries, sales representatives, computer operators
4	Self employed
5	Skilled: electricians, plumbers, telephone fitters
6	Semi-skilled: assembly-line workers, lorry-drivers
7	Unskilled: labourers, waitresses, cleaners
8	Underclass: long-term unemployed and sick

Source: Rose and O'Reilly (1997)

Constructs

An extension of Weber's notion that humans give meaning to their social world is the constructionist argument that there is no unadulterated objective reality. All physical objects and social phenomena are to a greater or lesser extent 'constructed'. They become 'real' when humans attach particular meanings to them.

From this point of view diseases are human constructions. They do not exist without someone recognising and defining them. Whereas the medical scientist believes that diseases actually exist and can be identified and described as 'facts', the constructionist argues that they only have the appearance of having a reality because of the coming together of certain historical and social processes. At other times, and in other places, they would either not be construed as real at all or they would be interpreted as different entities.

There is a link between 'cultural relativism' and constructionism. If all things (natural or social) are affected by socially produced values, then the worth of cultural practices other than our own cannot be judged on the basis of 'right' and 'wrong', or 'better' and 'worse'. Each culture can only be assessed in its own terms. We cannot declare that a set of beliefs and behaviours from another culture, no matter how virtuous or abhorrent they seem to us, merits either replicating in our culture or is in need of being extinguished within that culture.

Constructionism has been of major influence in theorising about criminality and deviance, including mental disorder, in the form of 'labelling theory' (or 'social reaction' theory). Labelling theory portrays 'crime', not in terms of the inherent biological or psychological characteristics of an individual malefactor, but as sets of actions or beliefs which are given the tag of 'deviancy' by the powerful in society (Lemert 1951; Becker 1963). What the labelling theorists argue is that an action is not in itself either 'normal' or 'deviant' until that meaning has been ascribed to it. That is, car-theft, burglary, or even murder, are not crimes until society (via its agencies of social control such as the police) declares them to be so.

Many 'crimes' are never categorised in this way because they have not been observed. People who carry out 'criminal' actions do not become 'criminals' if they are not caught and regarded as such. Moreover, large amounts of rule-breaking occur in society (for example, virtually all car drivers break laws concerning speeding, and perhaps the majority of young people have used illegal drugs or drunk alcohol under-age), but unless this is 'reacted to', it does not count as deviancy.

A distinction is made between primary and secondary stages of deviant labelling. Over a period of time an individual is socialised into a permanent deviant identity. That is, rule-breaking has only a negligible effect on how individual rule-breakers perceive themselves or are viewed by others. This is especially the case if our deviant actions go unnoticed by other people. But if our actions are uncovered, the reaction of others and the processes we go through as a consequence of being 'found out' can create a 'deviant career' (Goffman 1963). It is at this 'secondary' stage that the label starts to define the person, separating her or him from the rest of society.

The individual at this point becomes a fully fledged deviant, internalising the values that are associated with the form of deviance she or he has been labelled as deserving, and acting accordingly. The imposed label, therefore, manufactures the social phenomenon of criminality or deviancy.

Furthermore, the process of becoming a complete deviant is enhanced if the individual is clustered with people who have been given similar labels. 'Total institutions' such as gaols and asylums will reinforce a criminal or mad identity (Goffman 1961). The individual who is stigmatised by a deviant label becomes socially discredited and discreditable, and has her or his identity 'spoiled' by the reaction of the 'normals' (Goffman 1963).

The constructionist argument is not that all natural and social phenomena should be considered as 'made up' and treated as such. To recognise that everything around us emanates from particular viewpoints and beliefs is not to dismiss how 'real' these entities appear and feel. Humans construct their realities by objectifying subjective experience (Berger and Luckman 1967). Things such as steel, bricks, water, air, supermarkets, bicycles, grass, love, hate, intelligence and disease, are imbibed with pertinent and shared social meaning and utility. They therefore have a socially constructed vital capacity which overcomes the speciousness of their physical substance.

However, the ruminations of a disparate and perplexing band of thinkers, the post-modernists, have taken constructionism even further away from a belief in objective reality, to a point of extreme cultural relativity whereby everything can be 'deconstructed' and 'anything goes'. These theorists suggest that there has been a globalisation of cultural chaos, which began in the advanced capitalist societies but spread through mass electronic communications systems, and the internationalisation of business. The world is now characterised by a plurality of contending beliefs and packaged lifestyles (Crook et al. 1992). All aspects of social life (for example, health, holidays, sex, entertainment, leisure and housing) have become 'commodities'; and humans have been refashioned as 'consumers'.

Within such a pandemic cultural arrangement there can be no political, moral or epistemological knowledge that is regarded as superior to any other. The legitimacy of the 'grand narratives' (for example, nationhood, Christianity, Islam, Judaism, socialism, capitalism and science) that purported to explain the social, physical or spiritual world, has been supplanted. There has also been a demise in the degree of deference shown formerly to leaders, experts, teachers, the police and the judiciary, and the clergy. The old certainties have gone; truth of any sort is unobtainable; and ambiguity abounds.

We no longer have life-long careers, identifiable gender roles to follow, or consistency in what can be considered a normal family. We are just as likely to find solace in the ethereal publications of 'new-age' authors than we are in the sermons of priests. Visits to the health-food shop for a vial of aromatherapy oil or a bundle of herbs are as common as attendance at the general practitioner's surgery for a bottle of medicine or box of pills. Science and astrology are consulted for their prophetic explication on an equal footing.

Summary

The 'sociological imagination', supported by theories that examine social structure, the meaning individuals assign to their experiences and interactions with others, and the concreteness of their world, can contribute to the nurse's wider understanding of health, disease and the health-care system. That is, as Sam Porter (1998) explains, apart from supplying the nurse with a very necessary understanding of how social factors affect health and illness (the subject for the rest of this book), sociological theories can help to 'inform practice', and develop philosophies of care.

Further reading

Porter, S. (1998) *Social Theory and Nursing Practice*, Basingstoke: Macmillan.

Chapter 2

Health

> In our country today, too many people suffer from poor health. Too many people are ill for much of their lives. Too many people die too young from illnesses which are preventable. But at the same time, many people realise the value of better health.
>
> (British Prime Minister, Tony Blair, 1999)

What is health? Is a person healthy if she or he unknowingly has a tumour growing internally but regularly runs a marathon? At what point does that person stop being a 'runner' and become a 'terminally ill patient'? If my general practitioner, on the basis of a medical examination, informs me that I am healthy, but I 'feel' unwell, who is right? Can a low-caste child from the Indian sub-continent ever be described as healthy if she or he eats half the amount of food and lives for only two-thirds of the life span of a child born into a North American middle-class family? British citizens generally now live well into their seventies. Does this mean they are much healthier than British people were a hundred years ago, when most died much younger? Will it also mean that in one hundred years' time, when the British will on average live even longer, people today will be considered to have been unhealthy?

The difficulties in establishing a definition of 'health' are examined in this chapter. In tackling the question of 'what is health?', definitions of 'illness' and 'disease' need also to be discerned, as does the question of 'who is doing the defining?'.

Health polarities

Until relatively recently, the overriding interpretation of 'healthiness' was the absence of bodily or mental afflictions which either caused suffering to the individual concerned, incapacity in her or his daily activities, or were distressful to that person's family or community. That is, health has been for centuries defined negatively.

Furthermore, part of this negative interpretation of health centres on morality. Being unhealthy in both pre-industrial and modern societies carries with it an element of personal failure and a duty to become well (Blaxter 1990). To be unwell is a sign of inadequate will-power, even when disease transmission routes are unaffected by the most self-disciplined of individuals – gymnasts still do contract influenza, and runners can have heart attacks.

To some extent, all unhealthy people become socially excluded either permanently (as with chronic diseases such as AIDS and schizophrenia) or temporarily (as with most acute conditions). However, those who abstain from alcohol, cigarette smoking, unprotected sex and high fat and sugary foods do have the moral edge in today's health system. Indulging in these practices may attract social stigma, loss of employment and possibly the withdrawal of health-care services if patients are viewed by medical practitioners to be deliberately exposing themselves to 'unnecessary' risk.

Tribal healers, shamen and witchdoctors in pre-industrial socie-ties aimed to make their 'patient' well by removing malevolent spirits. For example, the traditional healers of the African Azande would suck from the body of a sufferer the 'evil pellets' thought to have been introduced into that person through witchcraft (Evans-Pritchard 1937). Hippocrates (c.460–c.377BC), using an approach which had its roots in ancient China and India, advocated the redressing of the balance between the four 'humours'. It was thought that these humours (black bile; yellow bile; blood; phlegm) were the essential constituents of the human body, and when in equilibrium a person was healthy, but when the balance was disturbed then pain and disease ensued.

The ancient Greeks of course did not have the benefit of x-rays, scanning technology or electron microscopes. Neither did they indulge in the surgical examination of either the living or the dead in a search for pathology. Although the second-century physician Galen (129–c.199) did study human anatomy, a comprehensive understanding of the workings of the body came much later. Dissecting human corpses became acceptable only in the sixteenth century; and it was not until the seventeenth century that the circulation of blood was outlined by the English royal physician, William Harvey (1578–1657). Thomas Sydenham (1624–1689), a self-taught medical practitioner, was to formulate a taxonomy of diseases, delineating such conditions as syphilis, measles, gout and dysentery. In doing so, he emphasised the objectivity of disease, separate from the sufferer. That is, the trend had been since ancient times to regard the individual and her or his state of health as integral, and to accept that there was essentially only one 'malady' that caused all symptoms. The implication from Sydenham's work was that people were susceptible to a variety of diseases, and that these could be described in detail, their origin found, and specific treatments offered.

Further objectification of disease occurred in the eighteenth and nineteenth centuries with the advent of a hospital system in Paris which was unprecedented in its size. This allowed for the easy observation and investigation of large numbers of patients. Moreover, the introduction into the French clinics of such apparatus as the stethoscope, invented by French physician René Laennec (1781–1826), contributed to medical practice looking deeper and deeper into the body for the causes and effects of diseases.

Michel Foucault (1973) uses the term *Le regard* (translated into English as 'the gaze') to describe the way in which particular groups in society view the world. Clinicians in the eighteenth and nineteenth century searched for the cause and effect of disease within the patient's (dead or alive) body. From then on, *Le regard* of the medical practitioner was becoming focused on the minute workings of the body, and in doing so was to lead to more control and regulation over what was to be considered 'normal' anatomy and physiology, and behaviour.

Whilst the stethoscope allowed the physician to search for specific signs of pathological change in the functioning of the lungs and heart in France, in Germany progress had been made in the operation of the microscope, devised originally in the eighteenth century. This led to further explanatory 'reductionism' as now individual cells could be observed, and conceived of as the building-blocks of human (and animal) life.

It was Rudolf Virchow (1812–1902) who then was to make the connection between changes in the composition and performance of cells and the existence of certain diseases. The effect of micro-organisms such as bacteria on tissues and cells was discovered by French chemist and biologist Louis Pasteur (1822–1895) and the

German scientist Robert Koch (1843–1910). These developments formed the foundation of scientific medicine.

However, whether health is viewed as being obtained through the calming of generalised disturbances, the excision of renegade spirits, or the curing of identifiable and localised rogue cells and microscopic pathogens, there has been a focus on 'malfunction'. More positive connotations of health, on the other hand, were being explored during the twentieth century. In particular, it was the World Health Organisation (WHO) which perpetuated an idealistic notion of health: 'a state of complete physical, mental and social well-being and not merely the absence of disease or infirmity ...' (WHO 1946). Moreover, WHO supported positive health in its 'Health For All', Alma Ata declaration in 1977, in which all member countries were entrusted to attain its capacious ideal (WHO 1978).

Governments give attention to both negative and positive definitions, but frequently, there is confusion over which is being targeted and which service should be used. For example, the vast majority of consultations carried out by general practitioners concern the presentation by patients of signs and symptoms from established ailments. Yet general practitioner surgeries are expected to be at the forefront of 'primary care' and preventative medicine. Moreover, despite the rhetoric of health promotion within the health services, most of the health budget is spent on curative medicine.

Furthermore, the rhetoric of positive health is advanced with great vigour not only in specific policies, but also by, for example, such agencies as the Commission of Health Improvement (CHI), which was set up by the Department of Health in 1999. The remit of this agency is the inspection of every hospital primary-care trust in Britain. Teams of doctors, nurses and other health professionals will review standards in each location, appraise how complaints have been tackled and assess patient satisfaction with the services they receive. CHI aims to ensure that up-to-date technologies are being used, cost-effective treatments are being prescribed and adequate screening techniques utilised, both generally and in particular cases such as cancer care. It also has the remit of reducing what the Department of Health describes as 'unacceptable variation in health provision' (DoH 1999a), and is supported by the National Institute for Clinical Excellence (NICE). NICE is a special health authority, also set up in 1999 by the New Labour government, and has the function of systematically appraising clinical interventions by health workers. Members of the institute's board will offer advice to the Department of Health and Welsh Assembly on the benefits and costs of existing and new medical and surgical treatments and technologies, as well as on health promotion policies (NICE 1999). However, such organisational innovations in the health service as CHI and NICE are primarily ensuring that 'illness' is being dealt with appropriately, rather than meeting the criteria for health as laid down by the WHO.

The New Labour government's health policy was enshrined in the White Paper *Saving Lives: Our Healthier Nation* (DoH 1999b). But the title of this document is in itself ambiguous and indicative of a Janus-faced health programme. That is, on the one hand 'Saving Lives' refers to the need to reduce early deaths from such diseases as cancer, coronary failure and stroke, as well as from accidents and suicide. On the other hand, 'Our Healthier Nation' implies an improved health status for each citizen. However, the placing of a colon between these two parts of the title suggests that the government believes that fewer early deaths can be linked to better health.

It may be that the politicians are not confused (except with respect to grammar), but utopian in that they claim to want to cure illness and upgrade the health of the nation:

> We [the New Labour government] want to:
>
> •   improve the health of *everyone*
>
> •   and the health of the *worst off* in particular.
>
> *Good health* is fundamental to all our lives. But too many people
>
> •   are ill for much of their lives
>
> •   die too young from preventable illness.
>
> (DoH 1999b: 1, emphases in the original)

But the government's apparent wish to solve all health problems does not produce a definition of health other than that associated with the lack of disease. For example, the Chief Medical Officer, Liam Donaldson, in the same document helpfully offers 'ten tips' for 'better health'. However, Donaldson's advice is very much geared to disease prevention rather than a 'state of complete well-being'. For example, he recommends a reduction in the amount of cigarettes smoked or stopping altogether, a diet rich in fruit and vegetables, increased physical exercise, attendance at screening clinics, if alcohol is consumed that this should be in moderation, protection from sunburn, the practice of safe sex and the management of stress through conversation and relaxation. All of these suggestions are geared towards impeding the onset of particular cancers and heart conditions, AIDS and psychiatric conditions. If the advice is followed (along with two additional tips: be safe on the roads; learn first aid) then it is conceivable that an individual will feel invigorated physically and mentally. But this will be a by-product of the government's fixed target of saving up to 300,000 (in England) 'untimely and unnecessary deaths' in ten years.

It was the seminal work of René Dubos (1959) that pointed to the fallacy of health as an ideal state. He argued that the idea of perfect contentment has been projected by many cultures throughout history. He refers, for example, to the ancient Greeks whose legends cited tribes living in distant parts of the world in blissful conditions, not working and not suffering from disease or infirmity. With reference to later civilisations, Dubos observes that the eighteenth-century philosopher Jean-Jacques Rousseau (1712–78) believed that the nearer humans were to nature, the healthier and happier they were. That is, for Rousseau humans became increasingly corrupted, both physically and mentally, the more 'civilised' they became. Today, a 'happiness industry' has been created comprising a disparate array of health-related faiths, including new-age philosophies, homeopathic potions, herbal remedies and various 'holistic' doctrines. Although very different from each other in terms of their attestations and techniques, all have the intention of combating the destabilising effects of modern-day life, achieving mind–body harmony in one way or another and getting closer to nature.

But for Dubos this search for a state of equilibrium between humans and the natural world is based on a false premise. Apart from for a few people, perhaps with the assistance of secular or religious indoctrination, mind-altering drugs such as alcohol, marijuana, or the 'better than well' personality change induced by such psycho-medication as Prozac, a condition of being at ease with nature is not possible. Nature is not a constant, resolute or benign entity. The delimitation of 'natural' events and phenomena from 'unnatural' on the basis that the latter refer to human activity and the former everything else is erroneous.

For example, before humans even came on the scene in the world, supposedly beginning the process of disrupting nature, the dinosaurs stomped around obliterating huge swathes of vegetation, killing other animals, or being prey to larger dinosaurs. Moreover, very suddenly they were wiped out by a cataclysmic event, quite probably involving meteors hitting the earth with such force that the resultant dust clouds thrown up into the atmosphere blocked out the sun's rays. Are these happenings any more 'natural' than the destruction of rainforests by South American and Tasmanian loggers, the killing of innocent civilians by the soldiers of countless numbers of countries, or the destruction of the ozone layer through the burning of fossil fuels in industrialised societies?

Furthermore, what is a 'natural' environment for humans? Is it the arctic wastelands? Could it be the 'red centre' of the Australian outback? Might it be the sunny beaches of a Caribbean island? Or are vibrant and well-serviced cities not more natural habitats for humans, as well as for a plethora of animal life and vegetation?

Moreover, there is a tension between individual happiness (in the sense of expressed and satisfied desires) and the common good. That is, the health of the individual may have to be sacrificed for the benefit of the health of society. Therefore, as Sigmund Freud (1930) was to argue, the basic ontological unease that humans have living in society can be seen as the consequence of successful social ties. For society to operate effectively, it is necessary to control aggressive and libidinous drives. This control, whilst having benefits for the individual (for example, to provide security), does produce negative consequences. Specifically, for Freud 'guilt' was an internalised mechanism generated by the moral standpoint of a particular culture in order to diminish the possibility of destructive (for society) hedonism.

Dubos argues also that the search by the profession of medicine for specific cures to specific diseases is based on another false premise. He suggests that the profession of medicine's quest to find solutions for all diseases is a 'hopeless pursuit' because most conditions are caused by a multitude of factors. Symptoms may be controlled, but, except for a notable few exceptions (for example, smallpox), medicine has failed to rid the world of most of the diseases it has been able to categorise. Moreover, even those it has previously controlled may not always remain dormant (for example, tuberculosis). Significantly, Dubos records that it was the very man who was to be so influential in the formulation of micro-biological explanations of disease, Rudolf Virchow, who also recognised social factors in the creation of epidemics. Virchow was not only a scientist but a social reformer who campaigned for action to be taken against poverty and overcrowding in order to prevent the spread of disease. Most infectious diseases have been made less virulent and less widespread through alterations to the social circumstances in which people live (better housing, safer working conditions, improved wages to buy more food) and sanitation and water supply, than by medical intervention. Medical practitioners, therefore, should provide individual treatment and support social change. This is the basis of much of the sociological critique of bio-medicine, and also the basis of 'social medicine'.

For Dubos, health is not contingent solely on biological and psychological qualities. Taking a relativist position, Dubos argues that true health is where individuals believe themselves to be healthy, and are viewed as such by their social group. There is not, therefore, a universally applicable state of healthiness. It is, implies Dubos, the very spirit of humanity, characterised by a never-ending search for excitement, acquisition and invention, that yields discontent. That is, a state of 'complete well-being' is unnatural for humans.

In order to substantiate the definition of health as the absence of disease (i.e. negatively) it has to be demonstrated that there are standard and universally applicable rules of human anatomy and physiology. That is, before we can know what is abnormal there has to be a concrete understanding of normality. For example, we cannot possibly diagnose someone's blood pressure as too high if there is not an accurate measurement of what it should be in the first place. To know that a cell is growing in a malignant fashion, there must initially be exact appreciation of how a cell grows usually. A precise acknowledgement of the functioning of the pancreas must precede the conclusion that a patient has diabetes mellitus.

However, there is no such guarantee of knowledge in all (and constructionists might argue, in any) areas of medical practice. Apart from doubts about certainty in diagnosis of even malignant cell growth, there are uncertainties over what is normal for the structure and workings of the whole of the human body (Davey and Seale 1996).

Lay health

Whilst health can be defined either as an ideal state or the absence of disease (and disease is what doctors describe), illness is the subjective experience of 'feeling' unwell:

> *Illness* can be taken to mean the experiences of disease, including the feelings relating to changes in bodily states and the consequences of having to bear that ailment; illness, therefore, relates to a way of being for the *individual concerned*.
>
> (Radley 1994: 3, emphases in the original)

Illness, therefore, is what the individual senses that is 'wrong' with her or him, and may lead to making an appointment to see a doctor. Disease is what the individual has wrong with her or him on the return from that appointment.

For the medical anthropologist Cecil Helman (1994), a wide variety of subjective evidence is involved in the process of defining oneself as ill. These perceived alterations can be in physiognomy (for example, loss or gain of weight), bodily emissions (for example, urinating frequently or diarrhoea), the working of specific organs (for example, heart beating fast or headaches), or the emotions (for example, depression or anxiety).

However, whether or not an illness is experienced in the first place, what meaning is attached to any pain or discomfort, the reaction the individual has to her or his illness, and the way in which both healers and society frame and respond to the individual, are all dependent upon the social context in which events are taking place:

> the same 'disease' (such as tuberculosis) or symptom (such as pain) may be interpreted completely differently by two individuals from different cultures, or social backgrounds, and in different contexts. And this will also affect their subsequent behaviour, and the sorts of treatment they will seek out.
>
> (Helman 1994: 107–8)

A ten-point inventory has been produced by David Mechanic (1968) of reasons why people proceed from feeling ill towards being diagnosed as diseased. An individual is more likely to visit her or his medical practitioner if one or more of her or his symptoms:

1 are highly visible and recognisable
2 are regarded as dangerous
3 disrupt working or social routines
4 occur repeatedly or persistently
5 are not tolerated due to a low-pain threshold or perceived offensiveness
6 are understood in terms of cause, treatment and prognosis
7 are feared greatly or alternatively feared only minimally
8 do figure high when compared with other priorities
9 are interpreted as associated with ill-health rather than with other 'normal' activities such as long working hours, bereavement, or physical exertion
10 can be treated easily in terms of available resources and time, and without embarrassment.

Hence, there are many psychological and social phases before becoming diagnosed as suffering from a particular medical condition. The process of becoming a patient (i.e. changing from 'being ill to 'being diseased') is not only dependent on the beliefs and actions of the individual, which in themselves are affected by social factors, but also upon the behaviour of health-care practitioners. For example, in my study of how people became the patients of mental health professionals (Morrall 1998b), I recorded how community psychiatric nurses (CPNs) act as gate-keepers for the psychiatric services. CPNs make decisions to attend general practitioners' surgeries on the basis of whether or not they need 'extra' patients on their caseloads, or at times to ensure that they retain good relationships with medical colleagues by taking 'difficult' patients off their hands. In doing so, they are regulating who does and who doesn't begin (or continue) a career as a mentally 'diseased' patient.

In the shaping of her or his recognition and appreciation of illness, the individual is interacting with her or his environment and significant others. Seeking medical help becomes merely one possible response to illness. In the vast majority of cases, however, medical attention is not sought when feeling ill. That is, most illness is dealt with by individuals themselves without any recourse to formal help from doctors or other health-care workers. A high proportion of the population has been reported as suffering from symptoms of illnesses which are not reported to medical practitioners. However, people may also suffer very debilitating symptoms (particularly mental problems) without attending a doctor's surgery (Morgan *et al.* 1985).

The term 'sickness' denotes the amalgamation of the two processes of being diagnosed as diseased and of feeling ill, and alludes to the existence of a social role when suffering from ill-health. It is society that confers particular behaviours onto an individual who has felt ill, and has been diagnosed as diseased by medical practitioners.

The WHO interpretation of 'health', as Aubrey Lewis (1953) has suggested, in being so all-encompassing and idealistic, is also meaningless. Moreover, those advocating such a definition miss the point that for most of the time both doctors and lay people conceptualise 'health' as merely the absence of disease. For Lewis an individual's belief that she or he is in good health (because she or he feels no pain or discomfort), is in marked contrast with the physicians' 'objective' diagnosis of disease using, for example, blood testing or scanning equipment. But the subjective vindication for feeling healthy is accomplished through the unconscious or conscious device of inspecting one's body and mind for disorder. Equally, the objective approach is to use medical instruments and knowledge to confirm or refute the actuality of ailments and injuries.

The importance of recognising lay definitions of health can lead to the suggestion that the only valid measurements of health and illness are those that are determined subjectively. Moreover, policy makers and practitioners need to recognise how health and illness beliefs of individuals vary between social groups and between different cultures. That is, relying only on 'objective' disease-based criteria for measuring health and illness is untenable.

Furthermore, medical and lay beliefs are not necessarily dichotomous ways of understanding health concerns. In most medical examinations, the patient's account of her of his illness is obtained and incorporated into the process of diagnosing disease. As Alan Radley (1994) notes, meanings about the significance of the symptoms are 'negotiated' in the doctor–patient encounter, and both condone what he calls the 'therapeutic illusion' whereby there is an acceptance (no matter how tenuous or contrived) of the efficacy of medical science. Where non-compliance (on behalf of the patient) occurs, this is as a result of an unresolvable clash between the lay and medical perspectives. The exceptions (i.e. when no negotiation can take place) are when an individual is unconscious as a result of an accident, or during surgery. Moreover, an individual's disquiet about, for example, a constant feeling of tiredness would in one way or another have been influenced by medical discourse which links lethargy to such conditions as iron deficiency anaemia or seasonal affective disorder. The person concerned may have read about the link between her or his symptom and condition in popular magazines, or watched a television programme containing details of new medical approaches in these areas.

Individuals themselves may have quite irreconcilable and fluctuating beliefs about health and illness. For example, they might give credence to a fatalistic perspective on developing lung cancer and continue to smoke. However, the same individual may attend a general practitioner's surgery asking for antibiotics to treat a septic wound. That is, on the one hand, irrefutable medical research into the cancer-smoking vinculum is denied, whilst scientific evidence of the effect on bacterial infection of systemic medication is accepted.

Lay conceptions of health and illness can also contain other dimensions that appear to be contradictory. Contrasting opinions between male and female notions of health have been observed by Mildred Blaxter (1990) in her 'health and lifestyle' survey. She comments that signs of physical fitness are important to both genders. However, amongst men (especially the young), physical fitness is related to strength and sport, whereas for women it is 'appearance' that figures highly in conceptions of health:

> When thinking of 'the healthy person', young men in particular stressed strength, athletic prowess, the ability to play sports. ... Women rarely mentioned sports or specific leisure pursuits. They did, however, frequently define physical fitness in terms of their physical appearance. They commonly mentioned being (or feeling) slim. To be fit [for women] was to have a clear complexion, bright eyes and shining hair.
>
> (Blaxter 1990: 24–5)

However, (younger) women also saw their health in terms of how good their relationships were with their family and friends, or in their (older women) availability to help and care for others.

It may be that an individual's expression of good health co-exists with obvious bodily dysfunction. For example, the loss of a limb or an eye may not prevent a person from believing that she or he is otherwise physically and mentally robust. Furthermore, there may be a reliance on a 'reserve' of health to carry a person through a period of illness (Herzlich 1973). That is, people may describe themselves as having 'good health' even when wracked by infection or in need of surgery to remove an excrescence. This store of health, it is assumed, can be called upon to defeat the disease or prevent others from occurring.

Social health

As has already been indicated above, there are social implications involved in the manifestation of health and disease. This is the case whether health and disease are considered real entities (the positivist position of the structuralists) or fallacious phenomena conjured up by medical and political discourses (the stance taken by constructionists). Expenditure on health care is enormous. For the year 1997 it has been calculated that $2,985,000,000,000 was spent globally on formal health-care systems (WHO 2000).

Friedrich Engels, co-collaborator of Karl Marx, wrote a social history of England's working classes in the winter of 1844–45. He described the appalling social conditions experienced by the poor living in the large industrial cities of that age. He also connected the cause of ill-health and mortality amongst the inhabitants of the slum areas, factory workers and the unemployed, to these social conditions. Engels' treatise is one of the earliest and richest accounts of how ill-health cannot be simply understood in terms of biology and pathology. In this extract Engels lays the blame for disease and death on the way in which (capitalist) society is structured, and in particular on the *bourgeoisie*:

> The manner in which the great multitude of the poor is treated by society today is revolting. They are drawn into large cities where they breathe a poorer atmosphere than in the country; they are relegated to districts which, by reasons of the method of construction, are worse ventilated than any others; they are deprived of all means of cleanliness, of water itself, since pipes are laid only when paid for, and the rivers are so polluted that they are useless for such purposes; they are obliged to throw all offal and garbage, all dirty water, often all disgusting drainage and excrement into the streets. ... They are given damp dwellings, cellar dens that are not waterproof from below, or garrets that leak from above. ... They are deprived of all enjoyments

except that of sexual indulgences and drunkenness, are worked every day to the point of complete exhaustion. ... How is it possible, under such conditions, for the lower class to be healthy and long-lived?

(Engels 1892: 129)

The circumstances in which the poor of the nineteenth century lived may seem to be no longer of relevance to the situation those living and working in urban regions have to contend with now. However, globally, the disagreeable side-effects of urbanisation and industrialisation affect vast numbers of city dwellers in developing countries. Throughout Africa, Asia, and in many parts of South America, poor people live in conditions as squalid as those found in London and Manchester 150 years ago. Whether it is the ghettos of Karachi, Cairo, Rio de Janeiro or Lagos, huge numbers of people live and die in vile conditions. Approximately three billion people in the world exist on less than two (US) dollars a day (Brundtland 2000).

At times the woes of the poor are made even worse by the deleterious results of corporate global expansion and related urban planning. An estimated ten million people, who are already living in an appalling environment and have grim health standards, are moved from their dwellings each year. One study of the Indian city of Mumbai (formerly named Bombay) by Emmel and D'Souza (1999) records how the systematic clearance of slum areas for new commercial and residential developments was, in the year 1998, responsible for the eviction of 167,000 people. One group of slum dwellers, who had been brought from their villages to work as labourers, were moved scores of times from their homes by demolition squads from land that had become valuable in the drive to modernise Mumbai. They now live in mangrove swamps reclaimed from the sea but which still become water-logged at high tide.

Emmel and D'Souza found evidence amongst the children of these slum dwellers of protracted nutritional deprivation, diarrhoea, respiratory disease and skin infections, which were linked to the transitory nature of their residence and the effect this has on the family finances:

Repeated eviction wears away at the household economy. Each time the huts were demolished, the women explained, money had to be found to rebuild the shelters. ... As one woman told us 'each time our hut is destroyed there is less money to feed the children. Who will feed the children?'

(Emmel and D'Souza 1999: 1118)

However, parallels can still be drawn between the predicament of the poor in England during its industrial heyday, and the way in which the underclass exist in the cities of post-industrial England. General practitioner John Collee wrote a regular column for *Observer Magazine* in the 1990s. In one of his articles he describes the situation he was confronted with daily in his surgery when working in a large English city. Many of Collee's patients lived in filthy and damp houses, were brutalised by their partners, had partners in prison or were mentally disturbed. Collee comments that with such patients, which he postulates make up the majority of those who attend the surgeries of general practitioners (if not the population overall), there is no point at all in treating specific medical complaints. He concludes:

we live in an unfair society. There is an enormous financial gulf between the rich and the poor which has steadily widened. ... We seem ... committed to preserving the social dung-heap, just as long as its crust remains firm enough to bear the weight of a privileged minority.

(Collee 1995)

It is not just the unfair structure of society, however, that works against the health of certain social groups, the vested interests of specific industrial enterprises can be paramount in how people can maintain their health. To a greater or lesser degree, governments have colluded with, or bowed to pressure from, owners of business and their shareholders, where there has been tension between health policy and profits.

Take the example of environmental pollution. Any proposals by local and national government to reduce the toxic outpouring from automobiles invariably meets with antagonism from the 'road lobby' (i.e. car manufacturers, haulage firms, large retailers and vehicle breakdown organisations). This means that each city inhabitant, with her or his five litre intake of air per minute, has no choice but to also inhale, in varying amounts, such pollutants as sulphur dioxide and lead (now on the decrease), carbon monoxide, nitrogen dioxide, ozone and sooty particulates.

Moreover, the death and injury tally on English roads alone, whilst less than most other European countries, is still startling. In 1997, 3,559 people were killed in road traffic accidents, 42,967 suffered serious injury and a further 280,978 slight injuries (DoH 1999b). Road traffic accidents are the biggest cause of accidental death amongst children. Each year nearly 400 children lose their lives as pedestrians, cyclists or car passengers. Action by governments and local authorities to makes roads safer for adults and children is always tempered by political and commercial interests which range from arguments about civil liberties (the right to own cars and drive without excessive restriction), to fears expressed by owners of inner-city commercial enterprises about loss of trade.

Bad diets cause ill-health; and food production and distribution are a matter of politics (Robertson *et al.* 1999). Moreover, Tom Marshall (2000) has described how the amount of illness-causing foodstuffs can be controlled through fiscal policies, and recommends tax disincentives on, for example, biscuits, butter, buns, cakes, puddings and ice cream. He suggests that the economic regulation of these high-cholesterol comestibles could reduce levels of ischaemic heart disease.

It has been suggested that the food industry has fought a 'rearguard action' to prevent the lowering of sodium chloride (salt) in their products (Woolf and Illman 1998). High levels of salt in processed food (used to preserve and enhance taste) have been linked to hypertension, cerebro-vascular disease, kidney failure, stomach cancer and osteoporosis. However, not only have sections of the food industry attempted to influence government health policies by lobbying politicians, but funds have gone towards research that then concluded there was no correlation between salt intake and some of these diseases.

But the most blatant attempts to undermine policies aimed at preventing serious disease have come from tobacco companies. Evidence of cigarette smoking being a source of lung cancer has been available for a long time, but has repeatedly been refuted by these companies. Paradoxically, and perhaps with an element of unforgivable cynicism, marketing strategies for cigarettes have included expensive and very public sponsorship deals with sporting activities. Commercial irony is perpetuated also in the forced display of health warnings on cigarette packaging. A number of these firms have allegedly deliberately masked these warnings by using the same colour of ink and typeface as the rest of the package (Browne

1999). But even if highly visible, the exhortation that 'Smoking Kills' is exhibited on a deadly product which is legal, sold openly, readily available and earns significant revenue for the government. Furthermore, as the sale of cigarettes has declined in the West, so the tobacco industry has turned its selling of these lethal products to developing countries, with one company accused of using the 'black-market': 'British American Tobacco condoned tax evasion and exploited the smuggling of billions of cigarettes in a global effort to boost sales and lure generations of new smokers, secret company documents reveal' (Maguire and Campbell 2000).

Susan Sontag's (1990) historical analysis of how conditions with unknown cause and ineffective treatment attract extraordinary levels of apprehension and disgust and/or romantic connotations demonstrates well the social context of disease. Sontag records that in the eighteenth century 'consumption' (i.e. pulmonary tuberculosis) became a symbol of gentility and vulnerability within the upper classes. Sufferers were viewed as having a 'sensitive' constitution. Internally, the disease was adorned as organic 'décor'. Externally, to appear 'consumptive' (pale and drained) was to be fashionable. To have the 'tubercular look' became a metaphor for exemplary breeding or a bohemian and artistic lifestyle.

By the mid nineteenth century, however, with the discovery of the responsible germ, the same disease had acquired a fearful reputation as an insidious contagion and indiscriminate killer of children and adults. Sufferers from the 'lower orders' in particular were considered to be morally and physically contagious, and consequently shunned by their communities. Cancer and AIDS were to replace tuberculosis as the mysterious, awesome and repugnant diseases of the twentieth century.

The pervasive occurrence of the self-diagnosed symptom of 'stress' as an indication or cause of disease can be viewed as the result of the chaotic world in which post-modern theorising indicates we now live. Stress, however, is only a problem if it produces the psychosomatic effect of 'anxiety', and thereby reduces the sufferer's ability to cope with her or his everyday activities. Most of us need some stress to be applied, by way of social expectations, in order to meet the demands of the workplace and responsibilities to dependent children, or simply to accomplish the routines of washing, dressing, cooking and interacting with other people. What the post-modernist proposition confers is the idea that the decay in regulated patterns of social behaviour and expectations has produced an epidemic of 'ontological insecurity'. That is, we no longer have any certainty about how to live out our lives, and have to make choices constantly about areas of our lives that previously were virtually set in stone. This induces a sense of psychological unease that may be reflected in the significant numbers of patients who attend doctors' surgeries because they are 'stressed'.

For example, changes to the role of women in society and their prominence in the workplace has created increased tensions for both women and men. Women are now faced not simply with a new role – that of paid worker – but with multiple roles as many continue to perform their child-rearing and housework responsibilities. Moreover, not only may the high suicide rate amongst young men be linked to a loss of the traditional 'bread-winning' role, but for both genders there is increased and prolonged apprehension about employment prospects in an economy that fluctuates habitually as each current technological innovation takes effect (Scase 1999).

Summary

The work of nursing has traditionally been concerned with disease. From the late twentieth century, the ideological focus of nursing work changed from addressing issues concerning disease, to that of health betterment. However, the concept of health is ambiguous, and this lack of clarity about what is meant by health is replicated in health policies. Moreover, an appreciation of what is meant by 'health' must include how ill-health is encountered and sensed by an individual sufferer, and how the social setting to which she or he belongs shapes such experiences.

Further reading

Aggleton, P. (2000) *Health*, London: Routledge, 2nd edn.

Chapter 3

Science

> In the sphere of thought, sober civilisation is roughly synonymous
> with science. But science unadulterated, is not satisfying; men
> need also passion and art and religion. Science may set limits to
> knowledge, but should not set limits to imagination.
>
> (Bertrand Russell 1961: 36)

Much of nursing and medical practice is predisposed to an
uncritical acceptance of science. Nursing and medicine (and all
other health-care disciplines) are engaged in the exposition of
scientific suppositions and methods to justify the care and
treatment that is dispatched to patients in the health service.
Research-based 'evidence' is given priority over other approaches to
understanding the patient's condition. The sociology of science,
however, aims to analyse critically the foundation of scientific
knowledge. At the core of this critique is the constructionist
proposition that knowledge of any sort, whether emerging from a
traditional source (for example, magic, witchcraft), co-existing lore
(such as alchemy, metaphysics, celestial prophecies, psychoanalysis,
paranormality, and religion), or science, is bound by temporality
and culture.

But, whilst superstitious beliefs may still be held by some people
in the West, and 'new-age' ways of viewing the world are growing in
popularity, scientific thought has become the predominant
epistemology, and therefore the most successful construct in
determining what is considered to be legitimate knowledge.
However, sociological thinking has challenged the authenticity of
the pre-eminent status of scientific knowledge. At its most
virulently post-modern, sociology claims that science is not factual

but simply one of many belief systems. That is, scientific knowledge is regarded as socially manufactured.

Positivism

Whilst the ancient Greeks viewed the gods of the planets as all powerful on earth, 'logical' thinking and political organisation, and 'rational' attempts to comprehend the origins of disease, were the precursors to the modern study of the natural and social world. As Bertrand Russell (1961) notes, the ancient Greeks were the inventors of philosophy, mathematics and science. Moreover, the Greeks did not separate philosophising from their accounts of natural events. The notion that scientific knowledge is a conglomeration of factual statements about real phenomena, and is therefore unhindered by theorising, is simplistic in the extreme. All statements of fact are mediated through theoretical conjecture. Natural laws (for example, gravity and the 'big bang') are speculations on the real world. All knowledge (whether scientific or not) succumbs to social processes in its production. It is not, however, inevitable to conclude from this that knowledge is fabricated totally, or that science is as good or bad in terms of an accurate exposé of reality as any other system of ideas.

In the 'irrational' Middle Ages, superstition and theology dominated as ways of comprehending humanity and nature. However, the rise of 'positivism' (defined as 'a means to understand the world based on science': Macionis and Plummer 1998) is attributed to the discoveries and inventions of a number of embryonic scientists.

In particular, Nicolaus Copernicus (1473–1543), a Polish mathematician and astronomer, was responsible for an account of the workings of the solar system which still holds today. Unlike the presiding belief since the ancient Greeks that the earth was the centre of the universe, the calculation of positions of the planets by Copernicus resulted in his pronouncement that the earth revolved around the sun.

The Italian physicist and astronomer Galileo Galilei (1564–1642) calculated that objects with unlike mass will fall at the same rate, and used the leaning tower of Pisa to demonstrate his theorem. His activities in astronomy (he designed an effective telescope) led to friction with the Roman Catholic Church. Galileo supported Copernicus' conclusion about the position and movement of the earth to other planets. He was forced by the interrogators of the

Inquisition to denounce his observations, and was placed under house arrest for the remaining years of his life, a span of a quarter of a century.

The Enlightenment philosophical movement of the eighteenth century in Europe brought with it new fervour in scientific development, and an 'age of reason' in which religious beliefs were questioned and individual equality and liberty pursued as human rights. Voltaire (1694–1778) campaigned irreverently in his plays against injustice, intolerance and bigotry, as well as stating his faith in science. Descartes (1596–1650) answered his own question 'how and what do I know?' with '*Cogito ego sum*' ('I think therefore I am'), declared that the mind was separate from the body, and contended that mathematics was the supreme scientific discipline. Isaac Newton (1642–1727), British mathematician and physicist, produced the laws of gravitational force, calculus, optics and motion, which were to lead to the classical scientific method of testing hypotheses with the view of deducing universal laws. By the nineteenth century, 'positivistic' science was offered as the sole and rightful exegetic paradigm for both the physical and the social world.

Gerard Delanty (1997) has catalogued the core tenets of positivism. These include:

1   all knowledge is susceptible to the techniques of natural science
2   'scienticism' – only scientific knowledge is credible
3   there is a reality which can be studied, and science stands ('objectively' and value-free) outside of this reality
4   empiricism – we only know what can be observed, and the experiment is the basis of scientific observation
5   internally coherent and universal laws exist which cross over bodies of knowledge and accord with the properties of reality.

So, for the positivist social scientist, society can be studied with the same principles and procedures as physics, chemistry and mathematics. There are, argues the positivist, cause and effect relationships between social phenomena. Just as mathematical formulae and the laws of physics allow us to predict how a car or rocket will perform, the science of sociology and anthropology can identify the origins of 'the family' and anticipate future patterns in human consanguinity.

However, despite the prominence of the scientific paradigm, surveys repeatedly show that the general public do not have intricate or even a basic comprehension of scientific rules and procedures (Fuller 1997). Science (and technology) may be the backdrop to much everyday human endeavour (for example, travelling by aeroplane, watching the television, switching on the washing machine, using the telephone), but people are not conscious of how it works. This lack of appreciation of what science is implies that the public's perception of its proficiency and applicability rests on a conviction not dissimilar to that adhered to by the medieval populace about devilry and the earth being flat.

Moreover, just as there are epistemological schisms between the study of the physical world and society, it is problematic to view the 'natural sciences' as a homogeneous enterprise. As Steve Fuller, Professor of Sociology and Social Policy at the University of Durham points out, physicists, chemists, mathematicians, palaeontologists and geneticists are exploring different – and frequently incompatible – domains. To transfer the rules and predictions of quantum mechanics into the study of fossils or DNA is perhaps in itself a fabricated, and therefore unscientific, process.

Steven Rose (1997), Professor of Biology at the Open University, goes further by illustrating how, within each scientific discipline, there are rival explanations of natural phenomena. He uses the allegory of five biologists enjoying a picnic by a lake when a frog jumps out of the water. This causes a discussion amongst them about how and why the frog can jump. Each biologist has a particular theory, all of which have been verified by extensive empirical observation.

First, the physiologist argues that the frog jumps as a direct consequence of the muscles in its legs contracting. These muscles are able to do so because of signals in the motor nerves of the frog's brain, which have originated from images of a nearby snake hitting the frog's retina. The second biologist, an ethologist, states that the physiologist has only explained *how* the frog jumped and not why. The frog has learned the behaviour of jumping away from predatory snakes in order not to be eaten (perhaps as a result of its own near encounters or from seeing other frogs being caught in this way). The third biologist, who studies development, suggests that the frog can jump because through its stages of growth (fertilised egg, tadpole, to mature frog) its nervous system has been 'wired up' in such a manner as to make jumping in these circumstances automatic.

Stepping into the debate, the fourth biologist, an evolutionist, claims that the frog jumps when in the vicinity of snakes because an evolutionary message, tied to its genetic make-up, has been passed down from its ancestors. Finally, the fifth picnicker, a molecular biologist, pronounces that all of the other explanations are wrong. To understand jumping frogs, we have to examine the minute details of the chemical properties of muscles and nerves, as this is where the biological events that mould such behaviours as jumping are taking place.

There is grand naivety in the positivist's assumption that science is 'objective'. What is studied, and how it is studied, depend to a large extent on whether or not funding is available, and funding depends upon whether or not particular organisations (such as drug companies, or government agencies) see commercial or political interests being met through the research. It is rare to find tobacco companies, breweries or the arms industry subsidising projects that aim to investigate the damage smoking and alcohol do to health, and the sale of guns does to life, unless the outcome may be to temper criticism of their business practices. Politicians are understandably wary of supporting research into, for example, new medical treatments if they envisage the public demand for a 'wonder cure' will outstrip the health-service budget. Moreover, researchers embarking on areas of interest that either do not require funding or attract financial sponsorship from organisations that do not stipulate preconditions (although will in the main still want the 'scientific method' to be adopted), are from the outset engaged in the subjective selection of their topic.

The process of disseminating research findings is projected by the scientific community as ensuring that only valid and reliable 'facts' contribute to authentic knowledge. Scientific discoveries are presented for objective and authoritative review in impartial academic journals. However, the editorial teams of academic journals, appointed in the opinion of the editor for their 'expertise' or as a consequence of personal associations, are themselves part of a scientific establishment that has preconceived interests and values with regard to what is and what isn't genuine scholarship. Furthermore, there is a hierarchy of credible journals, with pressure on researchers to publish only in those that are at or near the top of this hierarchy. Therefore, the subject and method of inquiry, and the medium of disclosure, is pre-given. Under these conditions it is exceptional for a dissenting author to be given the opportunity to be published.

Science is not even united over how to go about collecting and testing 'facts'. Karl Popper (1959), a philosopher with considerable influence on how science has come to be defined, argued for a specific procedure in the carrying out of science. Popper supported the testing of theory (or hypotheses) with the goal of 'falsifying' that theory.

For example, a nurse may recognise that listening to what patients say about their illnesses and circumstances appears to raise their self-esteem. The nurse may find that patients who suffer from a certain type of injury also report feeling a particular form of discomfort. She or he may detect that, in patients suffering from diabetes, drowsiness always accompanies hypoglycaemia.

The coming together of these sets of variables may happen so frequently for the nurse to induce that the respective variables are actually dependent upon one another (raised self-esteem on listening; discomfort on injury; drowsiness on hypoglycaemia). However, what cannot be claimed is that this will always occur. Just because a stone falls to earth at a certain speed when dropped from a tower, and does so thousands of times, does not guarantee that this will happen at every point in the future.

What Popper argued was that science should be embedded not in establishing constant truths – in his view an impossible objective – but in attempts to falsify correlations between events or phenomena (i.e. variables). Hypotheses should be formulated in such a way as to be receptive to being proven wrong. If they cannot be proven wrong, then this is bad science. In the case of the variables 'self-esteem' and 'listening', it is not enough (for Popper's brand of science) to say that they always appear together therefore they are connected to each other. The scientist has to set up an experiment which tests alternative suppositions. For example, the patients concerned could have their self-esteem measured before and after being listened to, and on other occasions where communication between them and nurses was prohibited. If self-esteem was demonstrated to have risen on occasions without any listening taking place the original assumption can be seen to have collapsed. However, although a finding that supports the link between listening and self-esteem would strengthen their assumed cause-and-effect relationship, this is only so for as long as it takes to assess the connection again using other hypotheses designed to falsify the original hypothesis.

This, for Popper, is how science proceeds. Each test of falsification either destroys a premise about the natural world, or allows it a stay of execution until a more lethal test can be devised. However, this view of scientific advancement was to be challenged by the iconoclastic claims of science historian Thomas Kuhn (1962).

Kuhn's contribution to a famous debate that ensued between Popper and himself was to project science and scientists as rather less than interested in the logical questioning of hypotheses on an unremitting journey towards truth – or at the very least travelling away from falsehoods. What Kuhn described were long periods of 'normal science' in which researchers simply accepted the presumptions of their predecessors. Scientists operated within an accepted paradigm, and for the most part did nothing more than address particular puzzles that were internal to that paradigm. Only those problems are researched, and conclusions sanctioned, that are 'plausible' within the principles of the paradigm. Any evidence that springs up during the 'normal science' that contradicts its precepts are dispensed with through ridicule or are contained by the setting up of theories that are in tune with the paradigm. But, at various times in the history of science, the build-up of evidence repudiating the accepted paradigm becomes so great that it starts to disintegrate, and an era of 'revolutionary science' ensues. The revolutionary period will be a time of turmoil in the scientific world, with much uncertainty and contention about what can be classified as authentic knowledge. At the end of the revolutionary interval, a new paradigm will emerge, and a period of 'normal science' will exist for as long as this paradigm can claim to explain natural, human or social phenomena. The new paradigm, however, is not any more 'rational' or 'developed' than previous views of the world.

For example, from the Kuhnian perspective, socio-environmental explanations of disease are being displaced by neo-evolutionary theorising, and research into genetic causation. Nursing, built on an epistemology of intuition and caring, has been replaced by the 'new brutalism' of evidence-based practice (Clarke 1999). It is probable, however, that the current acclaim of 'evidence-based practice' will reach its nemesis, and be substituted by a vogue knowledge-cult. Moreover, it may be that what post-modernists have identified as an age of cultural anarchy when all 'truths' are repudiated is really just a prolonged revolutionary era in the Kuhnian sense, and that eventually there will be a resolution to, and calming of, such epistemological strife.

The history of the discipline of sociology (and other social sciences) is declared openly as one of disagreement, political in-fighting, inconclusive theorising, inadequate empiricism, perpetual modification and occasional epistemological anarchy. Natural science has had a similar history, but tends to camouflage such commotion with a linear description of its progress. Science is portrayed as growing shakily but steadily towards uncovering more and more truths, until eventually a theory – backed by empirical evidence – will be procured to 'explain everything'.

Bio-medicine

The profession of medicine has an inexorable link with scientific positivism. The positivistic underpinnings of the natural sciences and technology have been used by medicine as 'ideological ammunition' (Morgan et al. 1985) in the processes of medicalisation and professionalisation. That is, medicine piggy-backs on the successes and promises of science. Science gives medicine credibility. This association with science has endorsed the status of medicine as a legitimate and valued profession, thereby allowing its practitioners to enter into many areas of human life formerly not their province. Nursing (or perhaps more accurately its elite stratum) also has a voracious propensity for self-glorification which an affiliation to science is deemed to promote. Through the digestion of scientific rules and techniques (whether conducting quantitative or qualitative studies) the leaders of nursing aim to satisfy their hunger for a profession ranking alongside that of medicine.

Medicine is not, however, mandated solely by science and technology (Seedhouse 1991). There are very different forms of knowledge and treatments within and across the various medical specialisms. Little common ground exists between the practices of the geriatric physician, the paediatrician, the micro-surgeon and the gene therapist. The trade of psychiatry uses talking therapies, justified through, for example, humanistic and cognitive-behavioural philosophies. But these intuitive techniques are incongruously juxtaposed with the scientifically sustained treatments of psychopharmacology and psychosurgery. Moreover, neither the talking therapies nor drugs and operations sit squarely, in philosophical or scientific terms, with electro-convulsant treatment, which has an inexplicable mode of efficacy.

But medicine is ultimately and vitally swayed by science, and scientific measurement and validation is projected as the ideal. Furthermore, medical practice has been seduced by an 'epidemic of techno-scientific discovery' which has taken place since the last quarter of the twentieth century (Nuland 1996). There have been revolutionary advances taking place in physics, chemistry, mathematics, computer technology, molecular and cell biology, and pharmacology, all of which medicine has devoured and proclaimed as its own. This is no more so than in the case of the human genome project. The scientific mapping of each human gene is anticipated to furnish medicine with cures for thousands of diseases. Just a few weeks before the beginning of the new millennium, one of the international teams working on the human genome project, announced that it had deciphered the first 33.5 million letter-code of chromosome 22 (Sanger Centre 1999). This was the first time any human chromosome had been charted. Although one of the smallest of the twenty-three human chromosomes to be found in each human cell, chromosome 22 is avowed to be associated with a throng of serious medical problems: schizophrenia; chronic myeloid leukaemia; miscarriage; congenital heart disease; some forms of learning disability; breast cancer; and cataracts (Radford 1999). This knowledge of the interrelationships between genes, behaviour, disease and the social and physical environment will be refined through the scientific collection and analysis of DNA and information about the habits and medical history of large population samples in a study proposed by the British Medical Research Council (MRC 2000).

However, the medical profession, even with the aid of a flourishing science, has still not actually conquered heart attacks, many cancers, strokes, AIDS or even the common cold. Despite improvements in treatment, the number of diabetes and asthma sufferers continues to grow; antibiotics are beginning to be considered a scourge because they are reducing the resistance of the population as a whole to disease; and pulmonary tuberculosis, malaria and cholera remain endemic in many parts of the world. Whilst pharmacologists and psychiatrists avow great achievements in tackling mental disorders, at best they are only alleviating symptoms. Moreover, the health of the poor in the industrialised world, whilst improved overall, has become worse relative to that of the rich, as has the health of the majority in developing countries compared to that of Western populations.

Professor Richard Smith, editor of the *British Medical Journal*, in a report of his speech at an annual conference of the Royal College of Psychiatrists (Boseley 1998b), acknowledged the poor scientific quality of medical knowledge. He stated that less than 5 per cent of articles from the 20,000 published medical journals worldwide are scientifically rigorous. The results of studies reported in these journals were often contradictory, biased, ungeneralisable, and some may also be fraudulent. He suggests 'evidence-based medicine' is likely to falter unless standards in research improve.

However, these deficiencies in the practice of medicine are counterbalanced by the well-publicised promise of future accomplishments which the new techno-scientific knowledge offers. Coinciding with reports of medical malpractice and ineffectiveness, stories abound in the media (and academic journals) about how medical science will provide cures for all cancers, every type of coronary failure and the full range of mental disorders, as well as preventing each inherited defect.

For example, on the same page of an edition of the *Guardian* (4 December 1999) newspaper two articles appeared. The first concerns a hospital where children had died and their internal organs had been removed by a pathologist for the purposes of medical research, but the parents had not been either asked their permission or informed of this procedure. The parents buried their children believing that the bodies were intact. One mother explains how a television programme into the affair had prompted her to contact the hospital. Ten years after her one-day-old son had died, she was informed by the hospital authorities about the organs that had been retained:

> I got a call from the hospital to tell me that [baby X's] heart had been removed. Then they listed other organs which had been removed, including his brain and organs from his chest and abdomen. ... I had basically buried my baby with very little left inside him.

This is a horrendous tale of unethical (and it has to be admitted, unofficial) medical practice. Furthermore, within the same story, reference is made to the medical malpractice that occurred at the Bristol Royal Infirmary cardiac unit where surgeons had been accused of incompetently carrying out surgery on babies with heart problems.

However, the second article is by contrast gratuitously triumphant about medicine's (potential) success in the field of cancer research:

> A revolutionary drug has been developed that appears to be capable of stopping leukaemia in its tracks ... Despite the small size of the study researchers say the findings may represent a genuine breakthrough in leukaemia treatment and possibly other cancers as well.

But the evidence-based movement in medicine and nursing is vulnerable to criticism for its reliance on the randomised control trial (RCT) as the gold-standard of research methodology. RCTs involve supplying one group of people a drug, surgical treatment, or psychotherapy while a placebo is given to another group. Neither group is aware of whether they are receiving real or spurious medical intervention. Responses from both groups are then compared, and possibly these are then compared with a 'control group' which has received no interventions at all. However, most trials conducted in this way have small samples, or are confined to particular groups of people (for example, patients in one or two hospitals, or self-selecting volunteers). Therefore, it is exceptional to be able to make generalisations to the whole of the population unless trials have been conducted repeatedly over a long period of time and in conjunction with other methods such as epidemiological studies.

Moreover, RCTs are based on a fundamentally defective statistical formula. Robert Mathews (1998) demonstrates that 'tests of significance', the very heart of scientific analysis, are actually based on a subjective assessment of probability. That is, the setting of the dividing line of '0.05 per cent' for evaluating the chance of an outcome being caused by an identified phenomenon was chosen in 1925 by Ronald Aylmer Fisher (who had attempted to correct a fault in a previous statistical theorem formulated by Thomas Bayes) because it was 'convenient'. The consequence of this arbitrary calculation of what is and what isn't significant is to exaggerate the importance of findings and produce false justifications for accepting highly implausible conclusions. This, argues Mathews, is why so many scientific and medical 'breakthroughs' discovered under experimental and/or laboratory conditions do not perform as such when in general circulation, and why there are so many contradictory results from studies examining the same problem. One study tells us not to eat butter, whereas a subsequent one indicates that eating butter will do us no more harm than eating margarine. One study suggests that drinking red wine is actually healthy, a second study that any type of alcoholic drink is health-enriching, and then a third that all alcohol should be avoided. These research flukes, for Mathews, are the result of the flaws in science.

Hence, conclusions from research trials cannot be held as infallible realities. However, it is somewhat disingenuous to accuse scientists of making such affirmations. The results of testing hypotheses in scientific publications are usually couched in tentative terms. The media not scientists announce that red wine, meat, margarine, coffee or tea can cure disease, and at some time later inform the public that these products are too dangerous to consume even in moderate amounts. The public, understandably, are not interested in deciphering complex research reports, but take an overall impression from what is being presented. This leads to facile interpretations of research outcomes. Scientists are well used to not declaring causal pathways between, for example, cholesterol and fatty foods, but to speculate on what the 'associations' might be between these substances. The media and the public, however, infrequently discriminate between 'causality' and 'correlation'.

Realism

To critique positivistic science, however, is not to necessarily follow Paul Feyerabend's (1975) route that 'anything goes' with respect to method. The methods of science have to be seen for what they are (inexact), and influenced by extraneous (social) factors. But the acknowledgement of uncertainty in science is not the same as arguing that science is worthless.

The presentation of science as defective, and therefore frequently misleading in its interpretation of the social and natural realms, should not lead automatically to the conclusion that these realms can be better elucidated by alternative epistemologies, or cannot ever be explained.

Indeed, the social-science perspective of 'realism' attempts to address the questions of what is knowledge?, and to what extent do social processes interfere with our ability to unearth reality? From the realist standpoint, human actors are shaped by, and assist in the shaping of, the social and natural world. That is, humans have a reflexive relationship with society and 'facts'. What an individual does and thinks affects the way in which society is structured, and what comes to be accepted as 'reality'. Equally, society and the natural world configure the circumstances through which human actions and cognition operate. Therefore, the 'human condition', the social system and 'scientific fact' are dynamic. Consequently, prediction (the cardinal goal of science) of human behaviour, social trends and natural events becomes difficult. These reflexive processes, however, do not mean, as the post-modernist would have it, that there are no facts, or that so-called 'facts' are so heavily laden with social meaning as to be devoid of any essential existence.

Realists accept that knowledge of what is a 'fact' can only be approximated. Such illnesses or syndromes as schizophrenia, autism, hypertension, migraine, cancer and obesity, may appear to constructionist sociologists to be 'disease fictions' because of the inability of the medical profession to be lucid in deciding their parameters. General practitioners may overuse such euphemistic diagnostic categories as 'viral infection' when unsure about symptoms, and may prescribe placebos when unconfident about whether there is a disease present at all. However, these medically ambiguous situations can be considered the effect of imperfections in scientific procedures, which are themselves the consequence of the interplay between human actors, society and reality.

By rejecting the standard antithetical positions of positivism (searching for an objective reality) and constructionism (reality is the result of subjective interpretation), realism offers a 'third way' in epistemology. However, rather than going down the post-modernist path of epistemological nihilism, whereby all knowledge is susceptible to deconstruction and all human action is (relatively) meaningful to individuals, groups and cultures, but has also no 'essential' meaning, realism reinterprets human understanding of the material and social world. That is, the relationship between epistemology (how we know what we know) and ontology (what we consider we are as humans) is redefined as having both objective and subjective qualities (Morrow 1994). Scientific methods can offer (some) insights into what we understand our existence to be, but human intuition, introspection and experience contribute also to 'knowledge'.

It is the realism of Roy Bhaskar that has produced an amalgamation of 'factual' and 'constructed' knowledge:

> men in their social activity produce knowledge which is a social product much like any other, which is no more independent of its production and the men who produce it than motor cars, armchairs or books, which has its own craftsmen, technicians, publicists, standards and skills, and which is not less subject to change than any other commodity. This is one side of 'knowledge'. The other is that knowledge is '*of* ' things which are not produced by men at all: the specific gravity of mercury, the process of electrolysis, the mechanism of light propagation. None of these 'objects of knowledge' depend upon human activity. If men ceased to exist sound would continue to travel and heavy bodies to fall to the earth in exactly the same way …
>
> (Bhaskar 1998: 16, emphasis in the original)

For Bhaskar, what we experience as objective reality can be viewed as contingent upon the relative values of our cultural and temporal existence. This does not mean that concrete realities are not all around us. However, we are, according to Bhaskar, restricted in our ability to know these realities because of the inevitable limitations imposed on us by culturally bound beliefs, and the socially contaminated (and hence inept) methods used by science to detect objective realities. Put simply, there are real objects and universal laws in our world, but humans can only experience these subjectively, and therefore can never 'know' in the purest sense, anything. Science offers us a 'best guess' of what these objects are and how the world is.

The continuous rearranging and updating of scientific knowledge (and at times complete paradigm-shifts in the Kuhnian sense), and the frequent publishing of contrary research findings, can be seen to be a consequence of the trouble humans have identifying accurately the causes of physical and social phenomena. Cognitive mechanisms and cultural norms and patterns 'mystify' reality – but, for Bhaskar, there is actually a reality to be mystified!

Bhaskar argues that 'intransitive knowledge' (i.e. invariable 'facts' that exist with or without our knowledge of them) can only be mediated through 'transitive knowledge' (i.e. the vocabulary, concepts and technologies of the 'science' of the day). Scientific endeavour is about investigating and attempting to disclose the real structures, processes, mechanisms and events of the world, through the use of understandings and prognostications that have been socially assembled over a period of time.

Contemporary conceptualisations of disease have been fashioned by the production of medical taxonomies, technologies and procedures over hundreds if not thousands of years. For example, the discovery of how blood flows around the human body by the English physician William Harvey (1578–1657) required the adoption of a conception of hydraulics that had been handed down from Greco-Roman civilisation. Today we utilise Harvey's 'physics' model of circulation to explain how nutrients are delivered to tissues, and infections and cancers spread to various corporeal sites, and how the body's defence apparatus is galvanised to fight these invasions.

Such a model is couched in transitive understandings. That is, this is the way in which modern Western-orientated societies have selected to appreciate aspects of physiological functioning, and is conducive to other styles of cultural representation in these societies. What is intransitive, however, are the primary constituents of the model, the underlying realities of the human body, its need for nutrients, its susceptibility to disease, and its capability to confront pathogens.

Brian Goodwin, Professor of Biology at the Open University in Britain, sets out the realist position on science neatly by asking and answering two incisive and interrelated interrogatives. He suggests that the answer to the query 'is there an objective world to be studied?' is no. Although there most definitely is a 'real world', the study of it is hampered by the researcher's entanglement in it. Any knowledge of this actual world, to a greater or lesser degree, will be an interpretation of real events. Therefore, the answer to the question 'is scientific knowledge a social construct?' is yes. Science is performed by humans, and is a social phenomenon. As such, its rules and loci are prejudiced by subjective reasoning and social processes. Scientific knowledge is an approximation of the objective world.

However, society functions relatively well in the province of this approximated reality. Most of us live for most of the time purposefully and effectively in this part-virtual world, unaware that what we embrace as substance is somewhat precarious. It would seem that we have an indelible craving to conjure up a solid world of matter, to 'make sense' of the complexities we perceive surround us, despite spasmodic insights into the contradictions and paradoxes that affect our social and natural world. We are in the main instinctive pragmatists, with only post-modernists engaged in the excavation of established perceptions of reality with the express intention of increasing rather than pacifying our epistemological and ontological insecurities.

The realist approach offers a rectified account of what the scientific endeavour is capable of, without needing to follow the 'nothing is real' mantra of post-modernism. Perversely, it is post-modernism that has been deconstructed by scientists.

Richard Dawkins (1994), the pre-eminent zoologist, biological determinist and author of 'popular science', accepts that sociologists have a point when they affirm that scientists are influenced by their social environment. He cites the example of Darwin having probably been inspired by Victorian values when he studied the evolution of animal and human species. But for Dawkins this does not mean that Darwin's theory of evolution is not correct. There is, argues Dawkins, something 'deeply silly' about the submission from (post-modern) sociologists that there are no facts. He asks for the following conundrum to be pondered over by sociologists:

> When you take a 747 to an international convention of Sociologists ... the reason you arrive in one piece is that a lot of western-trained scientists and engineers got their sums right. If it gives you satisfaction to say that the theory of aerodynamics is a social construct that is your privilege, but why do you then entrust your air-travel plans to a Boeing rather than a magic carpet?
>
> (Dawkins 1994)

Alan Sokal (Professor of Physics at New York University) and Jean Bricmont (Professor of Theoretical Physics at the University of Louvain in Belgium) have provided an irredeemable dismantling of the credibility of post-modern practices and conjecture. Sokal and Bricmont (1998) argue convincingly that post-modernists have misread and mistreated many scientific propositions. They attack the cerebral posturing and blatant academic dishonesty of prominent post-modernists.

In particular, Sokal and Bricmont assail the core concept of post-modern philosophy, 'epistemological relativism'. Epistemological relativism is the view that science is only a 'narrative' (or 'discourse'). That is, science tells a story about the events that has gained high merit in society, but is no more accurate than any other story that could be told. They argue that to accept historical accounts or alternative versions of scientific universals such as the earth is spherical is absurd. If in other ages or in other cultures the earth is accredited with a flat, oblong, or triangular shape, this doesn't make it a valid proposition. To believe in medieval times that the plague could be offset through the use of special aromas, or that some women were witches, can be proven to be abject nonsense.

However, Sokal and Bricmont's triumph over the post-modernists was achieved not through rational debate, but through a spectacular hoax. It was Sokal who submitted a largely nonsensical 'post-modernist' article to a leading American cultural-studies journal (*Social Text*). Using the title 'Transgressing the Boundaries: Toward a Transformative Hermeneutics of Quantum Gravity', the article was presented by Sokal as upholding a constructionist stance on science. Moreover, what was presumably especially attractive for the editors of *Social Text* was that it had been written by a real scientist.

The article was replete with impressive quotations from distinguished French and American intellectuals; it contained hundreds of footnotes and references. Sokal's parody of post-modernist thinking, full of pseudo-scientific justification and illogical political rhetoric, was published as a genuine contribution to the journal.

In a follow-up to the spoof, Sokal and Bricmont describe post-modernists Jacques Lacan, Luce Irigaray, Bruno Latour, Gilles Deleuze and Jean Baudrillard, as 'intellectual impostures'. They arraign these theorists for abusing science. This abuse involves the inappropriate use of scientific terminology and concepts in their own published material. That is, expressions and ideas from science are planted in post-modern literature to convey authenticity, but are often used out of context thereby rendering them meaningless, or are offered without any empirical justification. Put bluntly, these social scientists don't seem to know much about what they are writing about. Sokal and Bricmont conclude that post-modernists should not study what they don't understand (i.e. science).

Summary

Nursing has gone in the direction of attempting to 'scientise' its practices. That is, science is looked upon as a way of sanctifying and purifying nursing routines, whether this is preventing pressure sores, managing pain or assessing which communications are best suited for the amelioration of psychosis. However, science, and what scientists project as evidence, should not be taken at face value. Science is implanted in a social context, and therefore, what is cast as 'real' must be assessed judiciously. Equally, any sociological theory that purports to have destroyed the scientific endeavour by asserting that society conjures up all 'facts' should be appraised realistically.

Further reading

Fuller, S. (1997) *Science*, Buckingham: Open University Press.

Chapter 4

Power

Nurses, doctors, other health-care professionals and patients all have and use power in their relationships with each other. Power, as a social and personal endowment of authority, mediates and controls these relationships. It is essential, therefore, to understand the nature of power in practitioner–patient associations, and in interactions between practitioners. Without such an understanding, power differentials in health care may either continue uncontested, and this may be to the detriment of a particular discipline (for example, nursing) or gender (i.e. women health-care workers), or can undermine the movement to empower consumers of health services (i.e. patients).

In this chapter there is first a review of what is meant by 'power' and 'control' in society. Second, the case study of the 'sick role', the classic exemplar of the power dynamic between health-care practitioners and patients, is evaluated. Third, a critical account of patient-empowerment is presented.

Social power

Power is a complex phenomenon, involving a multitude of interconnected factors existing on a variety of different levels. Moreover, power loci can shift as a consequence of personal, interpersonal and social change. The twenty-first century has inherited global political and economic instability from the previous century, therefore identifying and defining who is powerful and where power is located is problematic.

The power of an individual rests upon such personal factors as volition, knowledge and physical and intellectual capacities. An individual's power is affected also by the norms and mores of the institutions to which she or he belongs. For example, an employer may invest 'power' in an individual employee by assisting her or him to obtain educational or vocational qualifications, providing increased pecuniary reward, or offering promotion. Furthermore, the power of an individual will be harnessed or inflated depending upon which social groups she or he is associated with. These in turn will be affected by their command over resources (for example, residential or commercial property, technology and information), and the prestige they are awarded. In capitalist society, the connection between the ownership of such resources and social status is infallible.

French and Raven (1953) and Collins and Raven (1969) formulated a catalogue of power types. Here they identified a number of different sources of power which involve individuals and social groups:

1   Expert power: where we assume that someone has greater knowledge and skills than ourselves because of long-training or experience (for example, a cyber-surfer asking for advice from a computer technician/programmer; the school teacher imparting knowledge to her or his pupils; the nurse trained in diabetic care providing guidelines on what food to eat and what to avoid).
2   Coercive power: where physical control is exercised over others by an individual or omnipotent group, and when corporal punishment may be enacted in order to uphold that control (for example, a parent deciding to smack her or his child to stop 'naughty' behaviour; soldiers or paramilitary police confining demonstrators; psychiatric nurses using 'restraint' or 'seclusion' to subdue a violent patient).
3   Reward power: where emotional or tangible disbursements are offered to alter conduct (for example, nurses caring for people with learning disabilities may use 'praise' or 'tokens' to reward and therefore encourage the learning of a new skill).
4   Legitimate power: where it is accepted another person or group (for example, judges, police officers, medical practitioners) has the right to influence others, and this right has been ratified by a legitimate source (especially the government). Coercion may be used to uphold legitimate power. For example, doctors and nurses may, in special situations, have the legal authority to force-feed, incarcerate, or compel a patient to have treatment.

5   Referent power: where another person has attributes that we wish we had ourselves (for example, a student nurse may try to emulate the caring qualities of a ward sister she or he is working alongside).

6   Informational power: we live in an 'information age'. Access to knowledge is becoming increasingly valuable and accessible (especially via the Internet), and this may transform the non-expert into an expert (for example, organisations representing the interests of particular groups of patients may supply data on current or experimental treatments about which most doctors and nurses are unaware).

For Dowding (1996) power can be conceived of as either the relatively simple and direct ability to bring about an intended outcome ('power to'), or a sophisticated skill to make something happen indirectly ('power over'). Power exists, therefore, when an individual or social group behaves in such a way that will produce a change in another individual or collection of individuals. But what is crucial with regard to the exercise of power in interpersonal relationships and between social collectivities is the selfish motive, even if it is rationalised as being implemented for the other person's or group's benefit. Moreover, powerfulness is no better displayed than when it is opposed and opposition is subsequently overcome: '*Power* is the ability of individuals or groups to make their own interests or concerns count, even when others resist' (Giddens 1997: 338).

A psychiatric nurse has the legal power 'to' prevent a compulsorily detained patient (and under certain conditions, a voluntary patient) from leaving the hospital ward. This form of power can be enacted openly and crudely by locking the doors of the ward. A nurse working on a general medical ward may execute power 'over' a patient by covertly withholding or manipulating information about a treatment, in a similar way to the 'spin-doctoring' of statistics indulged in by politicians, so that a particular reaction is forthcoming. For example, the nurse may wish to play down the side-effects of a drug to ensure that the patient complies with a prescribed course of treatment.

However, powerfulness is accrued to a much greater extent when others acquiesce. For example, for a medical practitioner to be so dominant in the doctor–patient relationship the latter must adopt the very passive 'sick role'. But power can be challenged successfully, and thereby diminished or lost altogether. There has in contemporary Western society been a demise of deference to traditional expertise and authority. Politicians are not thought of as highly by the public as they once were, perhaps because of the vast amount of media interest they receive (through which their proclamations can be contested), and the exposure of corruption amongst their ranks. Lawyers, judges and the police are seen to not be as credible as a consequence of a notable failure by the criminal justice system to consistently convict the guilty and free the innocent. Civil rights groups and relatives may use the courts to overturn medical decisions, for example with regard to the switching off of ventilators where a patient is perceived by doctors and nurses to be clinically dead and beyond rehabilitation. Moreover, the enormous social and political upheavals in Eastern Europe, Yugoslavia, Indonesia and many countries of Africa, are examples of once stalwart social systems being dislocated and/or replaced.

Power in society can be conceptualised as either being configured or diffused (Waters 1994). For the structuralist, power is considered to be in the hands of those people who occupy the upper regions of a social system that is always in one way or another stratified and hierarchical. A number of social groups (for example, men, the rich and whites) will have more power than others (for example, women, the poor and blacks).

However, some structural theorists (particularly those of a Marxist persuasion) view power as centralised within one part of the social strata. Specifically, in capitalist societies, the State (through its representative institutions) has accumulated and consolidated power, and works tirelessly to retain its omnipotence. Moreover, the State is in collusion with the capitalist class, to maintain economic and ideological sovereignty over the rest of society.

The interests of the dominant *bourgeois* class, having gained ownership of industry and commerce, and supported by the State, permeate all social and political organisations, and human relationships. As Lukes (1974) has observed, the desires of the mass of the population (for example, to have washing machines, new cars, exotic holidays, and even 'good health'), far from being down to the free will of the individual, are fashioned by the capitalist class. We accept as 'normal' the work ethic, paid labour, material possession and the legitimacy of the social hierarchy – all of which are necessary for the survival of the capitalist system.

In this way, structuralist theory regards the State (government and political organisations; legal, health and educational institutions) as a conduit for the interests of the dominant class. However, as Nicos Poulantzas (1978) has pointed out, the connection between the State and those with economic power may at times appear antithetical. For example, a government may institute laws which ensure a basic wage for employees, against the wishes of employers. Businessmen and -women may object strongly to the level of taxation on their commercial activities.

However, the social system itself is not being dismantled in these circumstances as the essential values and practices of capitalism remain intact. Furthermore, whilst professionals such as doctors may not be aligned unequivocally with the dominant class, they (and their nursing co-collaborators) either directly or indirectly shore up the capitalist system through their association with the functions of the State.

On the other hand, power is regarded by post-modernists as amorphous, factionalised and pervasive throughout society. Power from this perspective can be held by many different groups (including medicine and nursing). But no one group maintains power constantly, and power is not focused in one segment of society (whether the State, or an economic class) indefinitely.

Power is enacted by a multitude of groups and organisations in society. The subjugation of the powerless in these circumstances is legitimised and reinforced essentially through the language and associated symbols of power ('discourse'). Various social assemblages (e.g. political parties, corporate business, academic disciplines, the professions), create their own discourse and regulatory procedures. Control over everyday life (behaviours, attitudes) is dispersed through formal agencies such as the police, but also by such people as teachers, social workers, counsellors, scientists, nurses, health visitors and midwives. Hence, power spreads throughout society as if carried by capillaries that permeate each and every tissue of social life.

Foucault (1971; 1973) explored how medical knowledge has been constructed to form an apparently authoritative perspective (or 'gaze'). He argues that each society and every power-laden social grouping at every historical period, has a unique claim to comprehend 'reality'. The way in which we have come to think and talk about our bodies is controlled by the concepts, theories and symbols that have been supplied by the 'reality' of the medical profession.

Doctors use language (for example, Latin names for diseases and medical jargon), imagery (for example, the white coat, sitting behind a large desk and adopting a formal manner), and technologies (for example, stethoscopes, sphygmomanometers, body scans, laboratory testing, psychological assessments and genetic screening) in the application of their power on patients. Ascertaining 'the patient's view' becomes a technique designed to furnish the doctor's influence over the patient rather than helping to empower the patient in her or his dealings with the doctor.

The medical discourse in turn is a reflection of what society has deemed to be of significance at that point in time. Asking patients about their exercise, smoking and drinking habits, and encouraging them to take more responsibility for their health is not simply an example of good medical and nursing practice. The health-care agenda is pre-set as a result of social, economic and political contingencies which act beneath the surface of user–professional encounters. Western ideas of health care are, for example, a consequence of such historical events as the Enlightenment and industrialisation. Events such as these have gradually shaped our understanding of what is valued in society away from religion and community responsibility, to an acceptance of the singularity and sanctity of the human 'body' (Brooks 1993).

What can, however, be seen to be characteristic of either the structuralist or post-modernist approach is the pivotal role of 'power' in the maintenance of the influence of high-prestige groups and the stability of society overall.

The State and its affiliated institutions of control regulate behaviour, and place those who aggravate society into one or more of a long list of deviant categories. Legal, political, religious, educational and medical institutions all assist in the preservation of 'acceptable' forms of behaviour.

Every form of human society indulges in measures of social supervision. Without 'order', in its broadest sense, there would be no society:

> It is a truism that all societies, including the most unjust, un-equal, disorganized and anomic ones, manifest certain struc-tured patterns of interaction and routine behaviour which we refer to in aggregate as 'social order'. Otherwise we would not call them societies.
>
> (Scheerer and Hess 1997: 105)

Threats to either the whole fabric of the social system, or to the people who have gained prestige, power and wealth within that system, are mollified by the organisations of social control.

Social systems are liable to internal change, for example, as a result of alterations in the status and influence of various groups. Moreover, external pressures, as a consequence, for example, of the globalisation of technologies and economies, may cause prolonged periods of turmoil in the cultural practices of a society. However, the foundations of most societies are intrinsically adaptable and durable. The structural fabric of society is only at risk of total disintegration when facing extraordinary circumstances such as civil war, invasion by a foreign power, or economic collapse.

Not only do social control measures protect society as a whole, but the insecurities of the individual, generated by the predicaments (ethical and otherwise) of everyday existence, are also assuaged. Anthony Giddens (1991) suggests that in the industrialised world there has been a 'sequestration' of unsettling experiences, including those of 'nature', death, sickness, sexuality, criminality and madness: 'the ontological security which modernity has purchased, on the level of day-to-day routines, depends on an institutional exclusion of social from fundamental existential issues which raise central moral dilemmas for human beings' (Giddens 1991: 156).

That is, the modern State has attempted to lessen the feelings of vulnerability people undergo, and thereby evade primary questions about the meaning of life which may spawn new ideologies and insurrection. Science tries to tame the physical environment; hospices are used to hide the dying; the bedroom is considered the only acceptable arena for eroticism; and the physically and mentally sick are contained in hospital or their own homes.

Coercion by the authorised agencies of control is reinforced substantially by a continuous stream of complex messages that emerge from those with whom we share our social existence (Mathews 1993). We are bombarded constantly with both overt and subliminal signs from significant others and casual acquaintances. These signs shape the ways in which we perform as social beings by either encouraging or inhibiting our behaviour. Informal sanctions include mockery, reprimands, praise and an array of non-verbal communications such as frowns, smiles, touches and violent blows. Therefore, we are socialised into adopting the dominant convictions and socially approved patterns of behaviour through fear of condemnation by social control agencies, and by affirmative and confrontative messages from members of our family, friends, colleagues, peers and many others who we come across in our daily activities of living.

Sick role

The functionalist Talcott Parsons (1951) argued effectively that being ill was not simply about how micro-organisms, neoplasms, disability or trauma affect the body. Illness itself was regarded by society, suggested Parsons, as a form of deviance, and being ill is as much, if not more, to do with following a socially accepted pattern of behaviour (in order to become 'normal' again) as it is about a disease process. That is, we may succumb to the physiological and psychological effects of disease, but it is society that determines whether or not we should give this any credence, and if so how we should then behave and think.

Illness for Parsons had to be regulated so that society is able to function properly. Too much illness amongst the working population would be dysfunctional for industry, and place too heavy a demand on health and welfare services. Put simply, society cannot afford to have too many people not working through illness. Therefore, there has to be a formula for allowing a certain amount of 'legitimate' sickness. But the level of sickness should not get beyond the point whereby businesses become uncompetitive; there are not enough health practitioners to look after the sick; the health system becomes overburdened; or the accumulation of sickness benefits results in a fiscal crisis.

This formula takes the shape of a social contract between the person who is ill and health-care practitioners (principally, the medical profession) who represent the interests of society as a whole. It is the responsibility of the medical profession, supported by the discipline of nursing, to use its power to control access to the sick role. The contract is reciprocal for society and the patient in that both are aided by the actions of the medical practitioner. Society runs more efficiently, and the sick person is given succour.

The specific way in which the contract operates is through certification. Although self-certification for the initial stage of a period of illness has become standard practice for employees in many industries, a doctor's permission to be away from work for any significant length of time is still mandatory. Nurses working in general practitioners' surgeries may be delegated some elements of this process, and therefore are also involved in deciding who is and who isn't legitimately sick.

When an individual is given permission by health practitioners to enter into the sick role, she or he is accorded a collection of social privileges, as well as being given a number of social obligations (see Table 4.1).

Table 4.1 The sick role

Rights of the sick person	Rights of the doctor
1. Exemption from performance of normal role obligations	1. Controls entry to sick role
2. Exemption of responsibility for her/his illness	2. Granted access to intimate physical and personal information
	3. Professional autonomy and dominance
Obligations of the sick person	*Obligations of the doctor*
1. Must be motivated to get well	1. Acts in accordance with the health needs of the patient
2. Seeks technical help (i.e. from the profession of medicine) and co-operates with her/his doctor	2. Follows the rules of professional conduct
	3. Uses a high degree of expertise and knowledge
	4. Remains objective and emotionally detached

Source: Parsons (1951)

The sick person is given the right to stay away from work, and has exemption from family responsibilities. That is, in a literal sense she or he can 'go to bed' and begin the process of recovery. Hence resting is not just about allowing the body time to recover from the impact of disease processes, but also symbolises that the individual is undergoing the social process of 'being sick'. Moreover, society confers on the individual the right of not being blamed for her or his sickness where this has been denoted as licit.

The sick person's duty is to assist in the smooth functioning of society, once she or he has been awarded these rights, by being motivated to get well. That is she or he must do everything possible to ensure that the illness is cured in the shortest possible time. Behaviour such as going for a walk in the rain to consume large quantities of alcohol following a diagnosis of pneumonia will be viewed as reneging on the contract, and social approbation could ensue. This may take the form of the offender being shunned by her or his friends and colleagues, the rescinding of sick certification by the medical practitioner, or disciplinary action being taken by the employer.

Medical practitioners also have a set of social privileges and burdens (see Table 4.1). To begin with the profession of medicine is awarded the right to be the paramount agency in controlling access to the sick role. That is, no other profession, governmental department or employer can intercede in the doctor's decision to pronounce an individual sick. Furthermore, the doctor is granted ingress to intimate details of an individual's personal life and body functioning. A doctor has unprecedented social licence to probe (metaphorically and literally) every aspect of the patient's psychological and physical make-up. The patient lays bare her or his organs to someone (the doctor) who may be a complete stranger, but who has been conferred by society the liberty to inspect all emotions and orifices. Nurses conventionally had, in their role of supporting medicine, the devolved right to penetrate the patient's soma and psyche. However, nursing of late has extended this right by unilaterally claiming, as part of a declared pledge to holistic and individualised care, a need to know everything about a patient's biological, social, psychological and spiritual history.

Another expectation for medicine is the granting of autonomy and dominance in the health-care field. Conferment of professional status to medicine, therefore, can be seen as socially utilitarian. It follows that any challenge to medicine's authority (for example, by nursing becoming more professionalised, or the installation of non-medical management in the health service by the government) could be dysfunctional for society. That is, if the profession of medicine is losing some of its power in the health-care system, then the contract with society becomes uneven, and therefore compensatory measures may need to be taken such as providing other rights.

The socially bestowed obligations of the medical profession are first, to always have the health interests of the patient at heart when delivering treatment. Second, that its members must adhere stringently to the profession's own guidelines on clinical practice. Third, that the training of a medical practitioner must be rigorous, of exceptional quality, and that a command of her or his speciality (whether, for example, surgery, paediatrics, psychiatry, or general medicine) must be maintained throughout that individual's career. Lastly, in her or his interactions with patients and assessment of their ailments, a doctor must remain true to the scientific endeavour by invoking an invariably impartial and impersonal demeanour.

It is important to recognise that Parsons was not suggesting that his depiction of the sick role was to found in every case of illness. Nor was he arguing that doctors and patients performed consistently in their respective roles. As with other sociologists from structuralist-functionalist traditions, he is making a generalised statement about how society and its institutions operate.

But there are still faults with Parsons' model. Realistically, many people are not able to take advantage of their rights when sick. Women who are in paid employment and become ill still tend to have to care for their children and hence cannot easily 'take to their beds'. Whilst Parsons' sick role may be an appropriate way of describing what occurs in acute illness, when people suffer from chronic illness it is less likely that their social obligations will be met. This is no more true than in the case of such potentially long-term conditions as depression or schizophrenia. It is symptomatic of these conditions that the sufferer will not be motivated to get well.

Moreover, certain diseases carry with them a high degree of social stigma (for example, gonorrhoea, AIDS, alcoholism and epilepsy). Here the individual *is* blamed for contracting the condition. That is, with these conditions the right not to be held accountable for contracting the illness is not afforded.

Medical practitioners also may not always be working directly for the benefit of their patients. On occasions patients may be unaware that they are undergoing trials for particular treatments, or are having a drug prescribed that has been prejudicially selected as a consequence of inducements given to their doctor from pharmaceutical companies. Governments (as is the case in Britain) may restrict what treatments can be used by medical practitioners, or force the use of 'generic' medications. Such policies place restrictions on what can be offered by doctors, and *ipso facto* patients cannot be said to be having their needs met on every occasion. Furthermore, although it can be argued that these are exceptional cases given the enormous number of medical interventions conducted every day, accounts of incompetence and misconduct by medical practitioners appear regularly in the media. Therefore, doctors are not infallible with respect to their skills and erudition, and nor can their fallibility any more be concealed under a cloak of professional mystique. The press, public and government are far more aware of the reality of medical practice than has ever been the case before. We have also become aware that occasionally a doctor not only fails to toil to improve the health of her or his patients, but goes as far as murdering them.

However, it is important to appreciate the remarkable contribution Parsons has made to our understanding of illness. We may consider today his account of how society lays out rules for illness behaviour and regard parts of his model as overstated or inapplicable. But prior to his thesis on the sick role in the 1950s, there was no well-mapped awareness of such an unlikely part of the human predicament (i.e. illness) being a social, as well as a 'natural', phenomenon.

An elaboration of Parsons' functionalist sick role typology was produced by Szasz and Hollender (1956). Here there were three possible variations to the doctor–patient relationship, two of which implied that the latter could have a much more vital role than projected by Parsons (see Table 4.2). To begin with however, Szasz and Hollender conceded that in certain health–disease predicaments, such as during surgery, when a patient is comatosed, has a systemic toxaemia, or is in a state of severe shock, her or his engagement in the treatment process will be unavoidably inert. In these conditions the power of the practitioner is absolute. However, for many complaints (for example, acute respiratory or genito-urinary infections) patients are involved in their treatment to the extent that they 'co-operate' with medical directions. This level of participation becomes balanced, however, with a number of chronic conditions where perhaps the practitioner is more willing to give up some of her or his control to the patient either because medical knowledge about the disease process is imprecise, or the efficacy of treatments uncertain (as in, for example, AIDS, Alzheimer's disease, chronic anxiety).

Table 4.2   Sick roles

Type of role adopted	Examples
Active–passive (doctor is active, patient is passive)	Patient is unconscious, psychotic, or toxaemic
Guidance–co-operation (doctor guides, patient co-operates)	Acute conditions with known aetiologies, treatments and prognoses
Mutual participation (doctor and patient negotiate openly)	Chronic conditions with indeterminate aetiologies, treatments and prognoses

Source: Szasz and Hollender (1956)

A material issue about any model depicting the communication process between practitioner and patient, however, is that most illness is not treated by the formal health system at all. People in the main self-medicate or allow symptoms to take their natural course towards resolution. Doctors and nurses have nothing whatsoever to do with the vast majority of illness experienced by the population. Furthermore, patients may give the impression of co-operating with medical advice, but deliberately reject, ignore or deviate from given guidelines. Alternatively, they may not follow the directives because they did not understand them in the first place.

Significantly, the degree to which a patient becomes active in her or his treatment may be dictated by the type of disease, but the social grouping of the sufferer is perhaps more crucial. Moreover, a patient's involvement in her or his treatment may be encouraged, and opinion better respected, if there is a cultural affiliation (for example, if both are white and middle-class) between doctor and patient (Freidson 1970).

Szasz and Hollender's model can be very useful for nurses, not just as a descriptive tool through which they can evaluate their own interactions with patients, but as a method of reflecting on what *should* be the form of communication for any particular patient. That is, nurses may use this simple typology in their planning of individualised care, choosing which communicative pattern is appropriate to which patient. Furthermore, the three elements can be regarded as stages in a hierarchy of communication, with the activity of the doctor or nurse diminishing, as the involvement of the patient in her or his own care increases.

Patient empowerment

Parsons' passive conceptualisation of the patient's role has been affected by movements generally to empower the citizen and specifically to encourage users of health services to be active in their relationships with practitioners.

Gibson (1991) traces the history of empowerment in the health system. He suggests that it was the WHO's focus on health promotion during the 1980s that sparked off an interest by policy makers and practitioners in assisting people to take more control over their own health needs and in the prevention of disease. For Gibson, empowerment has, however, two interconnecting elements. First there is a focus on the individuals improving the quality of their lives within the social context in which they exist. Second, there is the need to raise people's consciousness about the antecedents of disempowerment:

> In a broad sense, empowerment is a process by which people, organisations and communities gain mastery over their own lives ... empowerment entails a process of helping individuals develop a critical awareness of the root causes of their problems and a readiness to act on this awareness.
>
> (Gibson 1991: 354)

Gibson concludes that such a definition necessitates a radical paradigm shift in that full empowerment can only be achieved if health-care practitioners and relevant social institutions transform the ways in which they relate to patients.

Britain of the 1980s saw political rhetoric from the 'new right' directed towards what was perceived to be a 'form of association' in which there was too much state control over both industry and the citizen's everyday life. The pendulum, argued political theorists of this radical persuasion, had swung too far in favour of interference by governments and 'experts' at the level of the economic, social and personal. Famously, Margaret Thatcher, the British Conservative Prime Minister from 1979 to 1989, announced that there was no such entity as 'society'. Under her influence, and that of her successor John Major, policies were installed to re-establish an atomised, self-possessed and empowered citizen. The 'common good' became equated with individual success.

The political messages of the British 'New Labour' government, elected in 1997 under the leadership of Tony Blair, however, once again make explicit the bond individuals have with the community. The Labour government's search for a 'Third Way' in British politics, which mediates between the individualism of rampant monetarist economics and the social engineering of the 'nanny state', has entered all areas of social policy including that of education, crime and health. For example, this government was to argue that the state education system should encourage individuals to accept the moral obligations of citizenship, as well as such specific social duties as 'parenting' (Carvel 1998; Walker 1998).

Professor Anthony Giddens, in his book *The Third Way: The Renewal of Social Democracy* (1998), observes that there have been fundamental changes in world politics and economics (principally due to globalisation) which demand new social agreements. Using slogans such as 'no authority without democracy' and 'no rights without responsibilities', Giddens argues that there is a need for all in society (workers, employers and government) to form an alliance in order to 'help citizens pilot their way through the major revolutions of our time' (Giddens 1998: 64).

But, accepting that those at the bottom of the social hierarchy suffer much more from most of the major causes of premature death than those who belong to the higher classes, the Blair government has targeted both social structure and individual behaviour (DoH 1998c). That is, the new social contract involves, on the one side, citizens adopting preventative measures (eating healthy food; taking regular exercise; practising 'safe sex'; giving-up smoking; not abusing drugs; drinking alcohol in moderation), and on the other side, the government tackling the issue of 'social exclusion' (poverty; unemployment; homelessness) and poor environmental conditions (pollution; danger in the workplace; overcrowded living conditions).

Following a long tradition of interactionist approaches to practitioner–patient communication, Martin Johnson (1997) conducted an ethnographic study in which he operated as a participant observer in a general medical ward of a large metropolitan hospital. He noted how nurses use their labels in their interactions with patients to establish control. Such labels as 'too demanding' or 'a nice patient' conveyed meanings of popularity or unpopularity, and of 'worth'. These social judgements had the consequence, for Johnson, of disempowering patients, but had the positive outcome for nurses of helping them to deal with emotionally distressing aspects of their work.

The power nurses have in the patient–practitioner relationship has been acknowledged fully by the United Kingdom Central Council for Nursing, Midwifery and Health Visiting (UKCC). In response to growing evidence of nurses abusing their power, the UKCC (1999) issued guidelines to protect patients. Abuse is defined by the UKCC as a misuse of power whereby physical, emotional or financial harm is (knowingly) done to a patient. The UKCC highlights the vulnerability of all patients, and in doing so inadvertently underscored the fallacy of the 'empowered' consumer of health services. That is, for many of those who are ill and asking for medical attention, it is axiomatic that they are disempowered. Being ill means a loss of control over one's life in one way or another, and to a greater or lesser extent. Particular ailments and ages, however, expose the sufferer to exacerbated mistreatment:

> People are vulnerable whenever their health or usual function-ing is compromised. This vulnerability increases when they enter unfamiliar surroundings, situations or relationships. Although illness and disability at any age can make people vulnerable, some groups of clients are more vulnerable to abuse than others. Those who are physically frail or have mental health problems, people with learning disabilities and children all require special consideration, to protect them from abuse.
>
> (UKCC 1999: 3–4)

David Armstrong's (1984) historical illumination of the purpose of eliciting the 'patient's view' in medical practice is at variance with that which suggests empowerment is the inevitable outcome of patient activity in the consultation process. Patients have for hundreds of years been asked to provide details of their conditions and the circumstances in which these were contracted. Using Foucault's (1973) concept of the medical 'gaze', Armstrong suggests that from the late eighteenth century clinical examinations united the search for 'signs' of disease within malfunctioning organs with the invited expression of 'symptoms' which could lead to more accurate diagnosis. But for the most part the worth of signs eclipsed the value attributed to symptoms. The patient was asked to speak, listened to, but not heard beyond helping to confirm or repudiate the significance given to physical indications of disorder. Communicating with the patient was a form of interrogation through which the medical perspective not the patient's could be instituted. However, through the influence of psychiatry (and in particular Freud's belief that there was a direct connection between 'inner thoughts' and bodily manifestations of illness), by the mid twentieth century the 'patient's' view had become an essential element of the clinical examination. What the patient said had now become important for a diagnosis and as a measure of how the patient was coping with, or adjusting to, the illness. Moreover, the influence of psychiatry continued to affect doctor–patient encounters so that to 'talk' became part of the treatment within both psychological and physical medicine. However, far from liberating the patient from the dominance of medical perceptions of her or his health, the 'patient's view' entered the epistemological territory of the doctor. It became subsumed within the medical discourse, where, arguably, it remains today, expressive and at times volatile, but hardly ever dominating.

Summary

Power infiltrates all social situations and relationships, including those that involve patients, doctors and nurses. Power congregates, however, in parts of society. It may be largely expropriated by the State and a ruling elite, or grabbed by disparate collections of people.

Uncontrolled power can pervert society, encouraging the disavowal of human rights. But the exertion of power by the State and other social institutions is also indispensable for the perpetuation of society and the protection of vulnerable groups. Without significant control mechanisms, society would disintegrate, leaving only anarchy and barbarism.

Moreover, if the profession of medicine loses some or most of its power as a consequence of empowering health-consumers (through, for example, the installing of official patients' advocates and advisors: DoH 2000a) the social contract that is the 'sick role' may collapse. If Parsons is correct in his assessment of the functionality of the rights–obligations equilibrium for doctor and patient, and the expediency of medical control over sickness for society, then what could supplant this arrangement? It is to think the unthinkable to muse that the sick role may be irreplaceable, and that the policy of empowerment may be counter-productive for patients and society.

Further reading

Dowding, K. (1996) *Power*, Buckingham: Open University Press.

Chapter 5

Professions

Medicine is a profession, and nursing wants to be one. Why? In this chapter I examine the role of the professions in society, the historical and present-day position of medicine as a professional occupation, and the potential for nurses to be enshrined as fully fledged professionals. Within this evaluation is a recurrent theme that professionalisation for doctors is an occupational tactic, founded on the principle of self-interest, which has been extremely successful.

This tactic, however, whilst embraced enthusiastically by nursing (or at least the elite managerial and educational section of the discipline) has not been so useful in achieving leverage in the occupational division of labour as it has been for medicine. Indeed, it is the very existence of medicine as a profession that attenuates, if not thwarts, the ambition of nursing.

Professions

At the beginning of the twenty-first century, the Western world and its institutions are undergoing rapid change as a result of the globalisation of the capitalist market and communications technology. This has led Stephen Jones (1995) to suggest that the Western world's 'post-industrial' phase, where the large manufacturing base of the economy has been replaced by service industries and finance corporations (Bell 1973), has entered a new period of development, 'cybersociety'.

The professions as social organisations are also mutating. A multitude of occupations are asserting that they are professions. The well-established professions of law and medicine are having to change their previously secure relationships with the State, the consumer, other occupations and society in general.

But what is a profession? Early twentieth-century explanations of what constitutes a profession were dominated by two connected approaches, which were rooted in the functionalist sociology of Emile Durkheim. Durkheim (1957) regarded the professions as an impartial and socially cohesive force. For Durkheim, they moderated individualism in society by reinforcing organic solidarity. That is, society was fortified and operated more harmoniously as a consequence of the professions' apparent devotion to the welfare of the community.

The first of these two early approaches was concerned with what 'traits' the professions exhibited. Altruism, a specialised and exclusive body of knowledge, lengthy vocational training, monopoly over practice and self-regulation were perceived to be the trademarks of high-prestige occupations such as law and medicine (Carr-Saunders and Wilson 1933). The second approach is much more obviously functionalist. Here the professions are regarded as directly helping to maintain the social order. For example, Parsons (1951) argues that the profession of medicine reinforces social stability by controlling entry into the sick role. This regulatory performance by medicine benefits society (sick people are encouraged to get back to work as soon as possible, and the lazy are discouraged from taking time off work) and the individual (she or he receives expert assistance to retrieve good health). Both of these perspectives: 'rest on the tenet that professions possess some unique characteristics which set them apart from other occupations and play a positive and important role in the division of labour in society' (Saks 1995: 2).

The trait and the functionalist definitions of professions have been subject to much criticism. In particular, they appear to reflect what those who consider themselves to be professionals believe are the characteristics of a profession. Therefore, there is a strong element of self-justification in describing the professions in this way. Moreover, such definitions are teleological. That is, they explain the existence of professions in society by referring to the purposes these institutions serve in society. Such an interpretation of a profession is circular and sterile. Specifically, there is no account of how 'social power' is obtained and exercised by the professions (Johnson 1972). These critiques have demonstrated that inequalities and oppression in the wider society are replicated by the professionals (Hearn 1982; Witz 1992).

With reference to medicine, feminists have revealed the centrality of gender divisions both within and between the various health occupations:

> feminists have argued that in the process of upward mobility, the male-dominated professions gain control over and subordinate female-dominated occupations. This is most clearly demonstrated in medicine where the medical profession is male-dominated and where the process of achieving its dominant professional status, the female occupations of nursing, health visiting and midwifery were subordinated ...
>
> (Abbott and Wallace 1990: 3)

Marx (1971, orig. 1867), with his concentration on the relationship of social groups to the economy, was dismissive of the role of professions in capitalism because of their perceived subsidiary or 'transitional' role mainly due to their lack of direct involvement in the process of production. It has been left to neo-Marxists to analyse more fully the structural position of the professions. However, reflecting the ambiguous position in capitalist society of the professions, Marxist views are not consistent. For example, Navarro (1986) argues that professionals are aligned with the capitalist class, and therefore contribute to the exploitation of the *proletariat*, and benefit in terms of remuneration and status from performing as an agency of social control on behalf of the State. According to Navarro, medical practitioners are 'trustworthy representatives of the capitalist class. Doctors (and nurses) get sick people well thereby sending them back into the workplace in order to generate more profits for the *bourgeoisie*.

On the other hand, some Marxists regard the professions as being located structurally alongside the *proletariat* (Baran 1973) as they are not owners of industrial or commercial enterprises and rely (certainly in Britain) for the most part on a salary rather than a surplus value (profit) generated from capitalist activities. The work of most medical practitioners is indistinguishable, therefore, from that of most other workers in contemporary society. Whether 'physical labouring' or 'mental labouring' is involved, doctors, like computer operatives and road sweepers, are subjugated to capitalist conditions of toil.

However, unlike Marxist analysis of the professions, which emphasises in one way or another their structural relationships to the mode of production, the post-modernist perspective suggests that they are not aligned necessarily with any one social class. The power of professionals is much more localised. Post-modernist accounts of the professions have recruited into their analysis Foucault's (1967; 1973) concept of 'discursive practices' (i.e. the technologies, procedures and linguistic styles of a particular social group). These practices allow a social group to gain power over others.

For example, Nicholas Fox (1992) conducted a study of the techniques used by surgeons to maintain and propagate their power over other workers employed in surgical wards and operating theatres, and patients. In his deconstruction of what he describes as 'the enterprise of surgery' he observed how the practice of asepsis establishes the supreme position and importance of the surgeon:

> Asepsis acts not only as a bacteriological insurance, but also as a rhetorical marker. ... For surgeons to possess a legitimacy for what they do (and hence a status other than that of a butcher or barber), these markers are clearly important ...
>
> (Fox 1992: 128)

For Fox, aseptic procedures signified the authority of the surgeon in the micro-world of the hospital surgical arena. The rigid and time consuming sanitising procedures (involving the cleaning of floors, equipment and bodies), together with the specially prepared protective uniforms worn by the respective players (surgeons, nurses, technicians, patients), all contribute to the elevation of the surgeon to the social position of star performer with unique abilities.

However, it is the systematic theorising of Eliot Freidson (1970a; 1970b; 1988) which has produced a debacle of the trait and functionalist definitions of a profession. Freidson identified that the professions served primarily themselves rather than their patients or society, and that their power was used to guarantee privilege.

Freidson applied the interactionist perspective of Max Weber to the study of the professions. He argued successfully that the concentration on definitional issues had produced descriptive rather than analytical accounts of how professions operate. Genuine professionals have autonomy over their actions and dominate everyone else working in the same field. What Freidson accomplished was a reformulation of the question about professions. His case study was the profession of medicine.

Medicine

Freidson directed attention towards the use of social closure and occupational control by some occupations to achieve professional status. Doctors, for example, have gained elevated social prestige by restricting who can practice in what *it* designates as the medical forum. Moreover, this forum is expanding and many parts of our lives, that had previously involved no interventions from doctors, are being medicalised. Scientific scholarship is utilised tactically by medicine to substantiate its dominance.

For Freidson, the medical profession has been motivated far more by self-interest than by its proclaimed altruistic intentions. Medical practitioners have campaigned historically to ensure that they alone can carry out bodily examinations and surgical operations and prescribe medicines. They have fought off other contenders for these treatment-franchises, such as lay midwives, druggists and knife-wielding retailers, on the basis that only they have accumulated the necessary esoteric knowledge and skills. Their goal has been primarily political not humanitarian.

For Freidson, whilst any occupation can announce that it is a profession, only those that have been granted (by the State) self-regulation over how and where they practise can be regarded as true professions. The turning point for the legitimisation of medicine by the State as a profession was the Medical Registration Act of 1858. With this act there was an amalgamation of three occupational sets of practitioners, surgeons, apothecaries and physicians. The act was to enshrine a united medical profession as the official organisation with jurisdiction over disease (Morgan *et al.* 1985).

However, autonomy and dominance for medicine have not been absolute. There is little doubt that the influence of the Royal Colleges (for example, of Medicine, Surgery and General Practice), the British Medical Association and the General Medical Council over health practice and policy has grown since the nineteenth century. But today there are conspicuous signs of a retraction of medicine's autonomy and dominance. Haug (1973) predicted that a process of de-professionalisation will occur as a consequence of the rise in consumer scepticism about the efficacy of 'expert' services.

This will happen, for example, because of wider access to the knowledge that is the bedrock of professional authority. Literature and computer programmes relating to health and illness (for example, to diagnose illness and list possible treatments) allow members of non-professional groups entry into bodies of knowledge that were formerly only the province of the specialist. The Internet allows for the retrieval of colossal amounts of data on any medical subject. Furthermore, consumers have become more demanding and well informed, thereby narrowing the social distance between the patient and the medical practitioner (Hugman 1991). There is also a plethora of 'charters' aimed at underscoring the rights of the consumer.

The active service-user also challenges medical hegemony by consuming alternative health care provision (now widely available), such as acupuncture, homeopathy, osteopathy, chiropractice, hydrotherapy, relaxation, massage and aromatherapy. That is, the existence of health ideologies and practices outside the formal medical domain undermines the power of the profession of medicine. If an individual can visit a high-street health shop and buy herbs or minerals to 'cure' her or his arthritis, depression or haemorrhoids, then the doctor's mystique is somewhat diminished.

However, the medical discourse is flexible. The medical profession is gradually extending its influence over alternative medicine and consequently reducing the threat to its prestige from this source (Saks 1995). 'Alternative medicine' was re-construed first as 'complementary medicine', suggesting that there was reciprocity between the two treatment spheres, but that orthodox medicine was the foremost. In turn, however, complementary medicine has been subsumed by orthodox medicine, and collectively they have become 'integrated medicine' (Burne 2000). Medical practitioners now prescribe these analogous therapies, and may provide treatment themselves or employ someone within their surgery to do so. Within this framework, the treatments that had stood in opposition to orthodox medicine will become increasingly susceptible to the rules of bio-medical science (especially to the requirement of testing their efficacy through randomised controlled trials).

Furthermore, as Freidson (1994) has argued, medical knowledge is highly technical. Hence it may be easily accessed but not readily understood. What is also pertinent in the medical context is that the consumer is unlike any other service user. She or he is ill, perhaps in great pain and discomfort, and possibly physically and emotionally incapacitated. It is improbable, therefore, that she or he will be able to tackle the assumed command the doctor has of the health system and disease processes.

In reality this medical knowledge is not available to all. There is a 'cyber-underclass' – i.e. the significant proportion of the population who do not have the opportunity to gain the skills to use computer technology, or cannot afford to buy the necessary equipment. Moreover, these information systems will be susceptible to expropriation by the professionals, who will provide the databases for the non-experts to use. Information will become divided between 'legitimate' sources and 'illegitimate' sources. Doctors will respond only to the knowledge that they originate and control.

Furthermore, the public's awareness of illegitimate (i.e. that which is unsanctioned by the profession of medicine) health advice and products that can be ordered through the Internet is becoming heightened. For example, a report from a consumer organisation has warned about the claims made by producers of 'health gadgets' advertised on the Internet such as muscle-toning mechanisms, herbal sleeping tablets, plaque-removing toothbrushes, spot-preventing facial ionisers, hair-growth inhibitors, and magnetic healing patches (Boseley 1999b).

Authenticated 'cybermedicine' was established in 1999 when the official NHS Internet site was installed to answer patients' queries about their symptoms. Computer software packages, using medical data, offer advice on diagnosis and treatment, and whether or not a medical practitioner should be consulted or an ambulance called. Further developments will be 'live' consultations with nurses and doctors. Doctors are using new technologies such as 'tele-medicine' whereby close-circuit video links, digital telephone lines and the Internet combine to allow a diagnosis to be made by specialists who may work at the other end of the country to the patient or even abroad. The patient visits her or his local health clinic where any number of medical procedures can be organised and relayed to the relevant expert:

> Digital photographs of retinas, taken by special cameras to monitor diabetes, will be sent by phone to laboratories; Laparo-scopes – photographs of patients' organs taken from inside the body – will be converted into digital images for transmission; Electronic stethoscopes, for monitoring heart rhythms, and digital X-ray machines will hook up directly to specialist units;

Video links will relay images of skin problems to consultants; Blood tests for diabetes and other diseases will be sent via computer links; Liver and kidney problems will be diagnosed using digital scans sent down the line.

(Durham 1998)

Such a parade of equipment signifies to the patient that doctors are at the leading edge of technological progress. Unless an equivalent expert or the most irrepressible of consumers, the patient will adhere to her or his passive sick role, awe-struck and bewildered by the magic of modern medicine.

The self-regulation and therefore autonomy of the medical profession has been affected by a rescinding of State support during the 1990s. In Britain, the Medical (Professional Performance) Act of 1995 means that doctors can now be penalised (to the point of being struck off the medical register) for simply not being good at their job, rather than, as in the past, having injured, sexually assaulted or killed one or more of their patients.

By the end of the 1990s, the General Medical Council had accepted the principal of periodic review ('re-validation') to assess medical competence. The New Labour Government post-1997 followed up the principle of accountability advocated by the previous Conservative administration with the concept of 'clinical governance' (DoH 1997). Clinical governance is the setting out of standards of service to patients that must be achieved, and both NHS organisations and practitioners must be held accountable for maintaining these standards. The chief executives of NHS Trusts will have statutory responsibilities for the maintenance of standards overall. 'Quality', evidence-based practice and the dissemination of innovative and effective ideas became the focus of health care delivery rather than 'financial efficiency'. The way in which practitioners work would become more and more scrutinised. Staff, including doctors, will be encouraged to report failings in their own work in order to then have the health systems that may be to blame altered or further training, where thought necessary, offered. But, disciplinary action, and possible dismissal, will ensue for serious clinical failures where the individual has been identified as culpable.

Two national agencies have been established by the government to oversee the operation of clinical governance as well as clinical effectiveness: the National Institute for Clinical Excellence (NICE); the Commission for Health Improvement (CHI). These agencies are answerable to government for the way in which budgets are spent. A doctor may wish to provide a treatment, but could be stopped from doing so if it is considered inappropriately expensive by NICE and/or CHI.

It was during the 1990s that the profession of medicine attracted a stream of bad publicity about some of its members. This, it could be argued diminishes its status as a munificent and skilled organisation. Jess Cartner-Morley (1998) reviewed newspaper headlines over a period of only one month. The following incidents are example of the failures in medical practice that were reported: babies dying due to under-trained and overworked medical staff; a girl of eleven waking up during an operation to fix her broken leg; the number of complaints to the General Medical Council about doctors at an all time high; over £3 million being awarded to a boy whose faulty delivery at birth by an obstetrician allegedly caused his cerebral palsy; a gynaecologist being found guilty of 'serious professional misconduct' and struck off the medical register; a general practitioner also adjudged to have conducted a sexual affair with one of his patients being struck off the medical register.

It was during this period that serious doubt over the medical profession's altruistic pretensions hit the headlines – the case of Dr Harold Shipman. Shipman, a general practitioner, was found guilty in 1999 of murdering fifteen of his elderly patients, and suspected of killing scores more. A medical practitioner, therefore, was to become Britain's most prolific serial killer.

Such was the degree of 'doctor bashing' that there were calls for the GMC itself to be abolished due to its apparent failure to protect the public from incompetent and malevolent doctors (Eden 2000). The point was reached whereby the British Medical Association, the doctor's trade union, declared that the GMC was failing the profession (Brindle 2000), and the government announced in its overhaul of the NHS a move from a 'consultant-led' to a 'consultant-delivered' health system (DoH 2000a).

The proletarianisation thesis (Oppenheimer 1973; McKinlay and Stoeckle 1988) projects the view that professional work is becoming increasingly subjected to management control at the instigation of the State. Supporters of this approach believe the fate of all professions is downward social mobility. From the 1980s onwards in Britain, bureaucratic limitations on the authority of the medical profession stemmed from the introduction of general management into the NHS. The NHS, rather than being 'administrated' by civil servants and clinicians, became 'managed' by agents of change from outside the health-care system.

But, in reality neither further regulation of medical practice nor general management has annihilated medicine. The profession is more than capable of dealing with public humiliation and political intimidation. The 'medical imagination' is insuperable, and the effectiveness of medical propaganda indomitable. Medicine remains an occupation with a substantial power base despite infringements to its autonomy and dominance.

The medical establishment will embrace some of the measures aimed at overseeing practice far more strictly than has been the situation over the last couple of hundred years. However, whilst some outside 'interference' will be inescapable, internal adjustments will be made to demonstrate that the profession is willing to change and therefore does not require external supervision:

> Ever since the scandal at Bristol Royal Infirmary which did so much to undermine public confidence in hospital doctors, the college [Royal College of Surgeons] has been ready to put together rapid response teams. The Bristol tragedy – the high death rates among babies undergoing heart surgery at the hands of two surgeons – was hugely damaging and the college has been determined to prevent anything similar happening again.
>
> (Boseley 2000)

Furthermore, organisational changes in the NHS have reduced substantially the effect of de-professionalisation and proletarianisation. For example, the forming of Primary Care Groups will create 500 conglomerates of general practice services, with doctors holding huge budgets and employing a range of support staff including nurses and health visitors, and eventually operating as NHS Trusts (DoH 1997). Moreover, it would appear that the NHS is to once again have medical practitioners (and nurses) at the forefront of planning health care in Britain: '[The secretary of state for health] revealed that 15 doctors, senior nurses and NHS managers are to be invited to join a beefed-up NHS management board ...' (White 2000).

For Freidson (1994) the level of control the medical profession has over its own affairs relies upon perceptions of the cup as half empty or half full. The State, however, can decide not only to drain autonomy and dominance from a profession, but can also top it up with fortified authority.

Nursing

> [Is nursing] essentially a subordinate occupation. ... Or is it an autonomous profession like medicine?
>
> (Dingwall 1986: 27)

Rafferty (1996) observes that the vanguard of policy from the discipline of nursing has been explicitly about the arrogation of schemes cultivated by others. The profession of medicine, not unexpectedly given its proximity to nursing and its unquestionable occupational accomplishments, has been a particular target:

> nurse leaders and policy-makers borrowed ideas and action plans developed by groups and institutions that they perceived as being already successful. ... [N]urse reformers often adopted strategies pioneered by medical reformers. Indeed medicine's influence upon nursing extended beyond the clinical environment: it provided a model for emulation in the propagation of a populist professional politics ...
>
> (Rafferty 1996: 182)

Nursing's big idea was that if medicine was a profession then it could be too. Professionalisation became the only occupational route for nursing. Along with other health-care disciplines (for example, physiotherapy, pharmacy, occupational therapy, health visiting and midwifery), nursing has been attempting to achieve this objective on the basis not of Freidson's critique but the 'trait' theory of professional identity. Nurses assessed what the descriptors of a profession (particularly medicine) were, and then identified ways in which the absent characteristics could be accrued (Jolley 1989).

However, professionalisation has been regarded by nurses both as a technique to gain status, and also as a method of uncoupling the conventional superior–inferior relationship with their occupational mentors:

> By tradition nursing has been seen as a dependent occupation, the nurse being expected to be the ears and eyes of the doctor,

loyally carrying out instructions and faithfully reporting back. A nurse was expected to be 'punctual, good tempered, obedient, and loyal to all rules as the foundation of her work'. She must also remember 'what is due to authority' and 'must ever remember that discipline and obedience are the keynote to satisfactory and efficient work in life'.

(Wainwright 1994: 3)

The most important element in the drive for professionalism has been the advent in the 1980s of 'new nursing', fostered by the senior stratum of nursing containing nurse managers, teachers and policy makers (Salvage 1988; Smith 1993). In part, new nursing is based on changes in the way in which nurses are educated. For example, a radically altered syllabus for nurses undergoing state registration was introduced (i.e. 'Project 2000'), and virtually all of nurse education was shipped into universities by the end of the 1990s.

There were also epistemological modifications to what the practice of nursing entailed. Nursing was to swing away (temporarily) from bio-medicine, extending its knowledge reservoir to encompass selected and frequently contradictory particles of the natural and social sciences. Nurses commandeered the philosophies of 'eclecticism' and 'holism' to vindicate their addressing health and illness issues by any and all available means, and to support what was to become the models, process and theories of its intellectual culture. The protagonists of new nursing also clasped to their ideological bosom the notion of 'primary nursing', which entailed placing the needs of the patient at the centre of care rather than organising services around 'tasks' and medical instructions (Wainwright 1994).

In the following decades, new nursing, imported from the USA, spread rampantly. The theories of how nurses should give care and help in the healing of the ill were to appear in nursing curricula throughout Europe. However, Hugh McKenna comments on the dogmatic way new nursing was introduced into practice, and on its uncritical acceptance and imprudent application:

In most cases, and with very little understanding as to what they were, nursing theories were applied, often without question, to a wide range of patient care settings ... there is little research evidence pertaining to the application, let alone the evaluation of nursing theories.

(McKenna 1999: IX–X)

With such an inauspicious inauguration, the difference this reconceptualisation of nursing has made in health care is debatable, as is its contribution to the cause of professionalisation. Feminism has also been influential in altering the direction the discipline of nursing has been steered in. The basic proposition from feminists is that nursing has been subjected to medical dominance because nurses are mostly female and medicine, whilst no longer numerically mainly male, remains directed by men (Gamarnikow 1978). Moreover, the cultural norms of bureaucratic organisations tend to be built on qualities that complement male behaviour (particularly competitiveness). From this perspective, professionalisation is hindered due to the 'feminine' attributes associated with nursing, and the responsibilities that women in a patriarchal society still bear. To be 'caring' is to be inert in organisational politics, and to be a mother and wife is to be too busy to be an effective contestant in the battle for occupational supremacy. Nurses, therefore, are disadvantaged due to their gender identity, and their gender identity is constructed by a male-dominated society and a masculine-orientated health system.

The interactions between nurses and doctors may be ostensibly configured on gender power. But a number of authors have attempted to interpret what is happening underneath the obvious display of control by doctors and the seemingly docile role adopted by nurses.

Most famously, Stein (1967) examined how nurses engage in a communicative 'game' with doctors. Nurses play this game to increase the amount of influence they have over clinical decisions and hospital policies. Doctors participate in the game to help resolve predicaments over routines or treatments where they suspect nurses know what appropriate action to take. Stein observes that what always has to be avoided is an apparent challenge to the power relationship between the two groups: 'The cardinal rule in the game is that open disagreement between the players must be avoided at all costs' (Stein 1967: 110).

Nurses offer advice tentatively and tangentially to doctors. For example, nurses may indicate non-verbally what medical actions they agree or disagree with. They may raise the possibility of an alternative way of managing a patient in such a manner as to not appear to have been suggesting anything other than what the doctors themselves would have wanted. Moreover, doctors may elicit recommendations from nurses by oblique invitation. That is, the doctor does not wish to convey to the nurse the idea that the latter's opinion is of value, other than as an appendix to medical judgement.

Deidre Wicks (1999), using data from interviews she conducted with nurses and doctors in Australia, has attested to how gender continues to mediate nurse–doctor relations: 'gender enters into, constructs, negates and shapes a large proportion of what happens and how it happens on a typical hospital ward' (Wicks 1999: XIV). But, Wicks highlights the complexity of these interchanges, and further elements of game playing. For example, she suggests that nurses are constantly reinforcing and undermining the gender-basis of the relationship with doctors. That is, nurses indulge in passivity at times, but are also mobile in offsetting medical directives when they consider that these are not in the interests of the patients. Resistance to medical imperatives by nurses is particularly common with respect to practices concerning wound treatments, pain relief and care of the dying. This ambiguity in role performance occurs as a result of a clash between what Wicks describes as 'oppositional discourses'. However, for Wicks it is not the case that these oppositional discourses produce a distinctive dichotomous relationship between nurses and doctors. For example, there is the discourse of medical science, with its concentration on objectified knowledge. This discourse is most prominent today in how doctors conduct their work. But the precepts of science have steadily infiltrated nursing practice. Moreover, there is also within both nursing and medicine a latent 'bedside-healing' discourse, with a far greater focus on the patient as a 'person' and on 'caring' than happens within the scientific discourse.

These complexities do not, however, negate Freidson's verdict on what makes a profession. His analysis is an 'ideal typification' (Freidson 1994). He is commenting on the overall contingencies of the professions. Not all of the particularities that make up his model will be present in an identical fashion in every profession. Furthermore, there will be countervailing and intricate forces at work within all professions, as there will be for those groups that are attempting to professionalise.

However, as we have seen, for Freidson the criteria of autonomy and dominance are paramount. Social groups may strive to gain advantage in the ordering of the division of labour, but Freidson points out that the State must be involved in the creation of a 'legitimate' profession. That is, any occupation may embark on a crusade to reach the status of a profession. Long training may be embarked upon, public service philosophies expounded, cryptic concepts and enigmatic modes of practice cultivated, and autonomous and dominating properties may even be acquired. But these occupations are not professions because their professional conduct has not been endorsed formally.

Moreover, these traits have been obtained by these disciplines in a premeditated craving for professionalisation:

> the leaders of aspiring occupations, including nursing ... insist that their occupations do provide prolonged training in a set of special skills, including training in theory or abstract knowledge ... but their meaning is suspect because the content and length of training of an occupation, including abstract knowledge and theory, is frequently a product of the deliberate action of those who are trying to show that their occupation is a profession and should therefore be given autonomy.
>
> (Freidson 1988: 79–80)

The problem for nursing is that it has all too obviously set about organising its training and theories for the sole intention of gaining a higher location in society. That is, governments, the medical profession, the NHS management, the public, the media and patients, cannot have failed to notice the social position nursing wanted to occupy, and the vacuousness of its political rhetoric. Nursing has been too nakedly egotistical. It has warned its rivals and seniors of its expectations. Unlike the long-term clandestine and sophisticated contrivances of medicine, it has been naive in its frankness about its designs on power for its own sake. The 'game' tactics employed by nurses, rather than being a display of emerging power, exemplify the weak position of the discipline compared to medicine.

For sure, nursing has improved its occupational status, and continues to do so. Nurses now prescribe a limited number of medications, 'triage' patients (i.e. select who needs most urgent medical attention) in a variety of clinical settings, assist surgeons with minor operations, manage alone special 'nursing-led' hospital or community-based units; are at the forefront of answering patients' questions (for example, as 'NHS Direct' telephonists and Internet operatives); undertake a plethora of university degrees and skills-improving courses; and at times practise unfettered by the overseeing tendencies of bureaucrats and/or their medical colleagues.

Indeed there appears to be a political commitment to extend further the clinical work that may be carried out by nurses and for a 'blurring of roles' between doctors and nurses (DoH 2000a). At the opening of a modernised hospital Accident and Emergency department in London, the Prime Minister and Secretary of State for Health announced new plans for nurses working in this and similar clinical units:

> Nurse practitioners and nurse consultants will play a greater role in treating patients on arrival, rather than simply assessing them. They will have greater powers to request X-rays, blood tests, and other diagnostic procedures, to interpret the results, give medication and discharge patients.
>
> (DoH 2000b: 1)

However, most of these embellishments to the nurse's role are indicative of medical intrusion into nursing. That is, nurses are performing as junior doctors rather than professionalised nurses. Doctors are passing on (as they always have done) areas of their work they no longer wish to discharge themselves. Alternatively, the State (with the connivance of nursing's representative bodies such as the Royal College of Nursing) is attempting to deal with specific organisation difficulties in health care. This includes, the poor recruitment and retention of nurses, periodic fiscal crises in the health system that make the employment of medical practitioners too expensive, and the need to reduce the working hours of novice doctors.

Furthermore, just as there are forces at work to reduce the strength of the medical profession, there are contradictory processes in the practice of nursing that have contributed to its failure to professionalise. For example, the creation of Primary Care Groups in the NHS and the likelihood that general practitioners will command huge health budgets, means that doctors will become the employers of large numbers of nurses. As an employee, the nurse will be able to play games but will always be at risk of being thrown out of the game altogether (i.e. by being sacked).

Another development in the health system that has had a dramatic impact on the status of nursing is the inexorable upsurge in the numbers of unqualified workers. At the same time as nurses are doing the 'dirty work' of medicine, health-care assistants are doing the 'dirty work' of nursing. There will be at some point a need to determine just who are the doctors and who are the nurses.

The attempt by nurses to be autonomous and dominate an area of work is also affected detrimentally by pressures to provide a cost-effective health service with a high turnover of patients. Medical commitment to science contributes further to this reversal. Today most patients, as a consequence of medical developments, do not spend enough time in hospital for the principles of new nursing to be administered. Acting upon the patient's biological, psychological, social and spiritual needs is presumably problematic if she or he stays under the 'nursing gaze' for only a few hours. Discovering what such needs are may not even be possible during a stay in the modern and fast 'through-put' hospital, or the community visit.

Freidson (1988) is resolute that nursing can never be anything other than a 'semi-profession'. The knowledge base for nursing (despite the attempts of the advocates of new nursing) remains within the remit of the medical model.

As Smith observes, much of the nurse's work remains shaped and directed by medical imperatives:

> Although the organisation of nursing care in hospitals has become more patient-centred in line with the nursing process, many tasks and routines shaped by medical diagnosis and treatment are still apparent. These tasks and routines include doctor's rounds, diagnostic tests and therapies on and off the ward.
>
> (1993: 210)

Doctors are responsible ultimately for the diagnosis, treatment, admission and discharge, of 'their' patients in most clinical situations, and therefore wield much influence over nursing practice.

One final salient point about the social position of nursing is that of pay. In 1998 the maximum salary of a ward sister was approximately £25,000 per annum whereas the basic salary of a consultant medical practitioner was £45,000 rising to nearly £58,000 (Boseley 1998a). However, senior NHS-employed medical consultants, with

discretionary awards, could earn in that year a salary of £112,000.
The creation of more 'nurse practitioners' and 'nurse consultants'
by the New Labour government, and the awarding of above-
inflation pay rises, is unlikely to redress the remunerative deficit
between the profession of medicine and the discipline of nursing.

Summary

The professions, like all social organisations, are liable to mutation
as a consequence of major developments locally, nationally and
globally. There are competing theories that attempt to uncover what
the character of a profession is, what the motives of its practitioners
are, and what role it plays in society. I have intimated, however, that
'power' is at the core of a critical understanding of the professions.
Moreover, power is reified for the professions, as Elliot Freidson has
testified, in the high level of autonomy over a work zone, and the
capability of dominating other groups of workers that conduct their
business in that zone. Significantly, however, the status of an
occupation that may be autonomous and dominant is diminished if
the State does not ratify its power.

Using Freidson's approach, the profession of medicine can be
viewed as remaining powerful, and nursing seen as relatively
powerless. Doctors may blunder and murder, but they still are astute
in their political machinations and have science as a sturdy ally.
Nurses may concoct theories and engage in practices that they
consider to be nourishing occupational elevation, but they may be
the mistresses and masters of their own subordination by marching
willingly and triumphantly into the medical encampment.

Further reading

Wicks, D. (1999) *Nurses and Doctors at Work: Rethinking Professional
Boundaries*, Sydney: Allen and Unwin.

Chapter 6

Medicalisation

The medical profession is (still) powerful, and in part this power is reified through the dissemination into the public's consciousness of medical ideas and technologies. This in turn shapes views of what is normal and acceptable in terms of behaviour and health. From a constructionist perspective, medicine is fabricating reality to advance its own interests.

Whilst at times antagonistic towards the profession of medicine for what is considered to be undue interference in their own sphere of work, nurses reproduce medical constructs of psychological and physical dysfunction. Nurses may object to the paternalistic, patronising and arrogant ways of their medical colleagues, but essentially embrace and duplicate the medical discourse. Hence, where in this chapter the effect of the medical enterprise on society is noted, it should be taken for granted that nurses are co-conspirators with doctors in the *medicalisation* of society.

Moreover, the medical enterprise is not just made up of doctors and nurses (and other paramedical disciplines such as physiotherapy, occupational therapy, pharmacy and radiography), but also includes the industries that manufacture the accoutrements of medical practice. In particular, the pharmaceutical companies are vigorous in the promulgation of medical hegemony.

The spread of medical predilections does not merely benefit its perpetrators. The profession of medicine is given licence by the State to infiltrate the thoughts of the population, and conduct its affairs with (relative) impunity, because there is a reciprocal advantage for society – stability.

But purely bio-medical explanations of reality are being superseded by an overlapping system of constructing the world. The ideological and technological forces of medicine, the paramedical disciplines, pharmaceutical companies and health promotion movements, have combined with the industries of health, beauty, sport, fashion, advertising and entertainment, to create a mono- lithic, pervasive and self-serving doctrine that promulgates a conception of normality entirely on the basis of health.

Medicalisation

The medical profession, argues Irving Zola (1977) has become the 'repository of truth', whereby the opinions of doctors hold great sway not only over anti-social behaviour, but over the daily lives of the general population. For Zola, virtually all areas of our day-to- day activities have been infiltrated by medical representations of what is normal (health) and what is abnormal (ill-health). That is, our whole existence has become 'medicalised'.

Moreover, Zola suggests that the profession of medicine has displaced the influence of religion. Doctors are the secular priests of contemporary Western society, and nurses their impious curates. Sagacity is imparted to all who attend the church of medicine. Like the clergy of old, doctors do not restrict their advice to one slice of human experience, but minister to a whole array of their congrega- tion's needs. The clinic has become the equivalent of the confes- sional box where misdeeds of the body and mind are divulged, and the surgical table is the altar on which salvation from the wickedness of disease is sought.

Many 'deviant' behaviours have come under the gaze of the medical profession. The following series of hypothetical scenarios by Conrad and Schneider illustrates the point well:

> Consider the following situations: A woman rides a horse naked through the streets of Denver claiming to be Lady Godiva and after being apprehended by the authorities, is taken to a psychi- atric hospital and declared to be suffering a mental illness. A well-known surgeon in a Southwestern city performs a psycho- surgical operation on a young man who is prone to violent out- bursts. An Atlanta attorney, inclined to drinking sprees, is treated at a hospital clinic for his disease, alcoholism. A child in California brought to a pediatric clinic because of his disruptive behavior in school is labelled hyperactive and is prescribed meth- ylphenidate (Ritalin) for his disorder. A chronically over-weight Chicago housewife receives a surgical intestinal bypass operation

for her problem of obesity. Scientists at a New England medical center work on a million-dollar federal research grant to discover a heroin-blocking agent as a 'cure' for heroin addiction. What do these situations have in common? In all instances medical solutions are being sought for a variety of deviant behaviour or conditions ... the medicalization of deviance.

(Conrad and Schneider 1980: 28)

A huge variety of other social and personal phenomena are now administrated by the medical enterprise. Menstruation is no longer a natural if unwelcome 'curse', but a medical condition that can be regulated and possibly dispensed with altogether. Pre-menstrual tension is not a period of unavoidable hormonal imbalance, but a symptom that can be thwarted. A large body size is not merely a material and commonplace consequence of a great appreciation of food (which signifies wealth and high social status in some cultures), but a stigmatised ailment that may require such surgical interventions as liposuction and partial gastrectomy. Feeling tired and disinterested in all aspects of daily life, but especially work, is rescheduled as 'chronic fatigue syndrome', and can be treated with drugs or psychotherapy. Faulty routine working practices, which require improved employment regulations rather than medical interference, nevertheless attract such catch-all and teleological disease tags as 'repetitive strain injury'. Being drunk and feckless is no longer a lifestyle choice, albeit a self-destructive one, but 'alcoholism', for which the 'addict' can be hospitalised and have medication prescribed. Deformity is not the unfortunate by-product of birth or accidents, but an unacceptable aberration in a world which values perfection, and must be corrected. Similarly, cosmetic surgery aims to remove blemishes and ugliness. Naughty school children now have 'hyperactivity' or 'attention deficit syndrome'. Difficulties in writing (dyslexia) or speaking (dysphasia) are traced to specific abnormalities of brain-functioning. Murder is re-categorised as 'Munchausen's syndrome by proxy'. Claiming falsely to have been abused in childhood is not just the result of shoddy counselling, being a liar, or making honest mistakes in one's intimate history, but is 'false memory syndrome'. Having bombs drop on you, your family and your neighbours whilst under siege from some rampaging and merciless army, and thereby becoming scared witless, is not explained as 'understandable given the circumstances', but is given the medical epithet of 'complete mass conflict disorder'. Sex offending is not only a reprehensible criminal offence, but a treatable malefaction, with specialist psychiatric services entering the prison services to create 'therapeutic environments'. Being miserable, grumpy and slothful during the dark and cold days of winter is re-construed as 'seasonal affective disorder'.

Moreover, not only does medicine's imperialistic tendencies continue to colonise new areas of our lives, idiosyncratic diseases are regularly detected in the most unlikely of surroundings. For example, the runner gets 'jogger's nipple', the sweater-maker, 'knitter's finger', and the oriental food faddist, 'Chinese restaurant syndrome'.

Medicalisation has particularly affected women. For example, the course of how a woman's state of mind prior to menstruation became a fully fledged psychosomatic affliction is charted by Catherine Bennett:

> Menstruation always did have a scurvy reputation, what with blighting crops and souring milk, but it took 20th century science to discover that women could be possessed by evil spirits before their periods had even begun. In 1931, pre-menstrual days were found to be a time of tension and hostility. They deserved a name of their own: PMT [pre-menstrual tension]. In 1953 Dr Katharina Dalton ... spotted a multitude of new symptoms, and invented something better: Pre-menstrual Syndrome, or PMS. This majestical syndrome embraces clumsiness, amnesia, fatigue, depression, anxiety, mood-swings – 150 different symptoms! It can account for completely different states of mind: lethargic and energetic; lecherous and unresponsive ... PMS has been accepted as an excuse for shoplifting, arson and homicide.
>
> (Bennett 1998)

Cecil Helman, a medical anthropologist, notes how the menopause has been redefined since the nineteenth century. Up until that time, most women died before losing their reproductive capacity. The naturally occurring reduction of oestrogen levels in middle-aged women causes hot flushes, excess sweating at night and changes in the composition of bones and in vaginal secretions, which signify the end of the child-bearing potential. As life expectancy grew in the industrialised world, the menopause as a medical category became a feature of every woman's life. Urbanisation brought these symptoms within the grasp of the enlarging and hospital-based profession of medicine. Women were treated as though they were ill, rather than just going through 'the change' from fertility to infertility. Now the menopause in effect is regarded as a 'disease' by doctors throughout the Western world. Although not universally acclaimed by medical practitioners as necessary, 'hormone replacement therapy' has become a frequently prescribed medication to help many women cope with the physiological symptoms of the menopause.

Medical practitioner James Le Fanu (1997) points out that huge numbers of people are diagnosed as having what he describes as 'non-diseases', and that this is a growing phenomenon due principally to the expansion in health screening. For example, he argues that tens of thousands are classified as 'hypertensive', and are prescribed medication on that basis, as a result of a doctor at some time taking their blood pressure as part of a formal or *ad hoc* assessment of general health. He even suggests that a minority of women have been erroneously diagnosed as having breast cancer because a 'lump' has been detected and pathologists are likely to want to err on the side of caution. However, these women continue throughout their lives to suffer from the psychological distress that this diagnosis entails let alone the bodily disfigurement of any resultant radiological or surgical treatment. Le Fanu goes on to identify what he believes to be the most prevalent way in which non-diseases are concocted:

> Much the commonest sources of non-disease today are the routine biochemical tests to measure the level of chemicals such as uric acid or cholesterol in the blood or to assess the functioning of the thyroid gland. Back comes an 'abnormal' result from the lab and, hey presto, someone who is well suddenly acquires a non-disease such as myxoedema (an under-active thyroid) or hypercholesteraemia (excess of cholesterol) requiring medication for life.
>
> (Le Fanu 1997)

Not only may health screening be unjustified because it medicalises people who do not have a disease, but it may be ineffective in unearthing actual diseases. Contentiously, a study of previous Swedish trials into the efficacy of breast screening by mammography, concluded that there is no reliable evidence that this particular screening technique saves lives (Gotzshe and Olsen 2000). The researchers suggest that for every 1,000 women screened biennially over a twelve-year period, only one breast-cancer death was avoided. The death rate during the same period had increased by a factor of six.

Michael Stone (1998) observes that there have been more psychiatrists in the last fifty years than in all of the history of the discipline, and the discourse of psychiatric medicine has entered irreversibly into the culture of Western societies. That is, personal thoughts, behaviour, emotions and social values have been thoroughly 'psychiatrised'. This approach is a variant of what Thomas Szasz describes as the *medicalisation* of problems with living (1973; 1974). For Szasz, the familiar and recurrent events and difficulties of human life (for example, communicating effectively with others, finding work, managing our financial affairs and coping with bereavement) are not the business of the medical practitioner. Doctors have only a responsibility to deal with those issues that have an organic origin.

The psychiatrisation of human life was initiated through the use of psychological methods of treatment in Victorian times, and the 'talking therapies' have retained a significant role in the practice of psychiatry. However, physical methods of treatment have become far more prominent in the process of medicalising problems with living. Psychosurgery and insulin therapy were introduced in the 1930s and 1940s, and then in the 1950s anti-psychotic and anti-depressant drug treatments were discovered. Towards the end of the twentieth century further major developments occurred in medical diagnostic technology (for example, computerised axial tomography; magnetic resonance imaging; neuroimaging; photomicrography; positron emission tomography; and single photon emission tomography). At the same time, a new wave of psychotropic drugs, such as the selective serotonin re-uptake inhibitors (SSRIs), were being manufactured.

The most obvious example of the psychiatrisation of everyday life has been through the proliferation of the drug fluoxetine hydrochloride (Prozac). Prozac, the first SSRI, is prescribed for depression but has become, alongside the male-impotency drug Viagra, a principal 'lifestyle' remedy. That is, just as Viagra has been utilised to boost male sexual prowess (rather than merely to address sexual dysfunction), so Prozac has become a 'mind-altering' chemical used to combat the pressures and disappointments of ordinary human existence. Peter Kramer, an American professor of psychiatry, champions Prozac as a 'personality improver'. Just as Viagra is projected as providing men (and possibly women) with extravagant orgasms, Kramer argues that taking Prozac can make all of us feel 'better than well'. It is, for Kramer, part of 'cosmetic psycho-pharmacology'. However, unlike somatic cosmetic surgery, the SSRIs can be used not merely to restore elements of the human condition, but to metamorphose humanity altogether. Kramer highlights the transformative qualities of Prozac with anecdotal depositions from his own practice. The following extract refers to his patient 'Tess':

> Here was a patient whose usual method of functioning changed dramatically. She became socially capable, no longer a wall-flower but a social butterfly. Where once she had focused on obligation to others, now she was vivacious and fun loving. Before she had pined after men, now she dated them, enjoyed them. ...
>
> (Kramer 1994: 10–11)

Not only does scientific doctoring still prevail in the consciousness of the public as the most significant 'world view', but the most irresolute area of medicine – psychiatry – is being seduced by the lush trappings of the positivist paradigm. The individuation of health is increased through new technologies and drugs as the physician's 'gaze' once again centres on the internal organs of the patient. That is, the social and political environment is displaced as the search for 'disease' concentrates on the infinitesimal within the human body.

In the main sociologists have taken a very critical stance towards the process of *medicalisation*. The term itself is one invented by social commentators to describe how the medical profession has a negative effect on individuals and society. Apart from the obvious 'social control' aspects in medical practice (which sustain the *status quo* and therefore benefit the elites in society), there is an indirect 'control' effect of *medicalisation* that is far more potent.

Medicine, with science as its epistemological benefactor, individuates social problems through this process of *medicalisation*. This has the effect of reducing the obligation on the State to adjust any of the socio-environmental factors that may have produced what presents as the 'medical' problem of an individual.

When a doctor treats a patient for an ailment such as bronchitis, heart failure, lung cancer or mental disorder, the focus of the intervention is on the individual. It is the individual who is asked to strip for examination, it is her or his blood that is sent to the laboratory for investigation, and to that person medication is supplied or surgery administered. However, many (if not all) serious illnesses have social and environmental dimensions. The major killers are contingent upon poverty and bad housing, air-borne pollution and hazardous employment conditions. But it is not the workings of society that are exposed in the doctor's surgery, nor are its unsound framework and defective institutions transported to a social policy unit for academic appraisal, nor is it society that is revitalised with an injection of fairness or the excision of asperity.

By concentrating exclusively on the patient the medical practitioner is individualising social problems. That is, medical practice reinforces the very social system that is the source of much disease. Moreover, the responsibility of the State to change society is diminished whilst doctors carry out remedial interventions on individuals. But this is not without a high cost to the State. Although *medicalisation* assists in the maintenance of social stability, it is expensive. Unchecked, the pioneering ambitions of medical practitioners will produce more and more diseases to be detected and treated by a growing throng of advanced technologies.

However, the medical profession is being influenced to some degree by the new public health movements that provide a wider knowledge base for the determinants of health and illness (Davies and Macdonald 1998). Bio-medical and individualistic explanations for what maintains health and causes ill-health are being encapsulated within a more comprehensive and sophisticated explanatory framework which at least in part acknowledges socio-environmental factors.

Medicalisation, however, may be the consequence of not just the imperialistic drives of the medical profession with its concomitant function of social control adding impetus and legitimacy. As Scambler (1997) notes, in part medical hegemony is the result of its actual success in treating (some) diseases. Moreover, the prospect of huge medical advances due to genetic mapping, computer technology and the effect of drugs on human biochemistry gives medicine at least the prospect of further achievements. A realistic perspective accepts that medical progress is characterised by hyperbole and catastrophe, but this is only to be expected given the innate problems that science has in defining its terms of engagement. That is, science is only able to approximate real events, and scientific medicine only makes 'best guess' evaluations of the cause and therefore the treatment of disease. Moreover, both science and medicine are housed in social contexts that set and drive their respective and coupled agendas. However, no matter what faults there can be detected in scientific and medical endeavours, there is a general inclination towards the discovery of facts and cause and effect relationships. There will never be absolute knowledge, nor socially untarnished understandings of what makes up the physical and natural world and what exactly generates and cures all ill-health, but this should not lead to a discounting of what can be known. The mistake made by the constructionists (and those supporting the *medicalisation* thesis) is an old one – throwing the baby out with the bath water. To imply that there are social connotations to be taken into account in the way in which, for example, colonic cancer or schizophrenia is conceived, is reasonable. To deny the reality of the distress, pain and the accompanying bodily or psychological transmutations is both irresponsible and callous.

Furthermore, the *medicalisation* of certain conditions brings with it great advantages for the individual. Madness reformulated as a medical category, even if enforced treatment and incarceration ensue, is surely better for the sufferer than being burnt at the stake following a designation of 'witch'. The disruptive pupil may receive welcome and extra support at school if her or his parents ask for a medical diagnosis of hyperactivity.

In this sense the medical profession is not merely 'empire building' but is responding to consumer demands. Helman comments on menstruation and the menopause, two intrinsic episodes in womanhood that have been medicalised over a period of one generation, but which also have been covered by the medical epistemological umbrella at the demand of women themselves:

> In the case of both the pre-menstrual syndrome and menopause, it can be argued that two of the natural physiological events of women's lives have been redefined by some clinicians as 'endochrine deficiencies' or; 'diseases'. This 'medicalization' means that some women have become more dependent on the medical profession and its treatments than their mothers ever were. However ... many women have also welcomed the devel-

opment of those medical treatments that have relieved the
unpleasant symptoms of both menstruation and menopause.

(Helman 1994: 162)

But the consumer will only be able to demand products and
services, whether these be organic food, improved rail travel, in vitro
fertilisation, anti-depressive drugs, or hormone replacement
therapy, if an expectation is generated first by the respective
industries, or at least the possibility of such products and services
being available is placed (through advertising or debate) in the
public domain. A spiralling appetite for medical interventions,
therefore, is hatched from the self-serving asseverations of medical
research and the commercial interests of the pharmaceutical
industries.

Iatrogenesis

Increased medicalisation also means that the dangerous consequences of medical interventions will become more widespread. For
example, Abraham (1995) suggests that the testing and regulation of
pharmaceutical products remains far from satisfactory. Abraham
points out that the public is perpetually at risk from such medical
catastrophes as the 'thalidomide incident', whereby pregnant
women were given a 'safe' drug, which was then to cause severe
foetal deformities. The editor of the *Lancet*, Richard Horton, gives
warning that:

> drugs are licensed by government and marketed by industry
> well before they are proved safe. An alarmist claim? Only last
> month, Troglitazine, a drug launched in October [1997] and
> prescribed to 5,000 British diabetics (and with world sales of
> $137 million) was withdrawn from the UK by Glaxo Wellcome
> because it was worried about damaging side effects on the liver.
>
> (Horton 1998)

The impression of medical infallibility has been contrived by what
Ivan Illich (1977) describes as 'awe-inspiring medical technology'
and 'egalitarian rhetoric'. But, for Illich, the medical establishment
has put both the health of individuals and society in jeopardy as a
consequence of doctor-inflicted injuries and loss of self-autonomy.
This is what Illich describes as 'iatrogenesis' – i.e. illness, disability

and dependency that would not have occurred if doctors had avoided giving treatment.

Medical intervention, argues Illich, is such a cause of morbidity it can be viewed as one of the most rapidly spreading epidemics of modern times. The iatrogenic epidemic takes three forms. First, there is *clinical iatrogenesis*. Here Illich is referring to the straightforward and relatively immediate side-effects of medicines and operations. Second, there is *social iatrogenesis*, whereby the whole of society, as a consequence of *medicalisation*, becomes dependent on the medical profession. Doctors 'sponsor sickness' and concoct a 'morbid society' by stimulating demand for curative and preventative medicine.

> Social iatrogenesis is at work when health care is turned into a standardized item, a staple; when all suffering is 'hospitalized' and homes become inhospitable to birth, sickness, and death; when the language in which people could experience their bodies is turned into bureaucratic gobbledegook; or when suffering, mourning, and healing outside the patient role are labelled a form of deviance.
>
> (Illich 1977: 49)

People become 'addicted' not just to medicines but to the medical profession. Such dependency is what, for Illich, has made the medical profession extremely powerful.

Third, Illich argues that both *clinical iatrogenesis* and *social iatrogenesis* lead to such entrenchment of medical authority in all areas of human life that the individual loses her or his ability to make autonomous judgements. This end-product of medical intrusion into how we organise our lives Illich describes as *cultural iatrogenesis*. Whether it is about how to bring up our children, how to care for each other, whether or not we should work, how to grow old, how to procreate or have sex, what meaning can be attributed to our thoughts and behaviours, or how to die, doctors are consulted. Moreover, for Illich *cultural iatrogenesis* has incapacitated the individual to the point that she or he is unable to accept pain, suffering or death as an inescapable part of human existence. Being anguish-free is to be also free of reality, and therefore not fully human. Humans need discomfort and grief to be in touch with the natural world of which they are part:

The modern medical enterprise represents an endeavour to do for people what their genetic and cultural heritage formerly equipped them to do for themselves. Medical civilization is planned and organized to kill pain, to eliminate sickness, and to abolish the need for an art of suffering and of dying.

(Illich 1977: 138)

Illich recognises that negative effects of a physician's or surgeon's therapy have always occurred. Doctor-inflicted trauma has been the result of professional callousness, negligence and incompetence throughout the history of medicine. Indeed, at times such malpractice has been justified by the medical profession as the inevitable repercussion from administering untried treatments which in the long run will benefit humankind. That is, mistakes have to be made as part of the process of learning about what works and what doesn't in medical practice. However, he makes the point that as medical practice discovers more puissant treatments to fight otherwise untreatable diseases, so the sequela becomes all the more sinister.

The most vile period of immoral experimentation of this sort occurred during the Nazi rule in Germany, where doctors conducted trials on those who were unable to object to becoming guinea pigs in the plan to create a master race. However, clinical trials continue to be dangerous to the patients who participate in them with procedures for storing, administering and recording side-effects of the drugs being tested commonly ignored, and patients not being told of the risks or being asked to sign consent forms only in retrospect (Boseley 1999a). There are approximately 3,000 of these clinical trials each year in Britain, involving hundreds of thousands of patients. Serious breaches of protocol, if only in a minority of these tests, not only threaten the health of the participants, but undermine the credibility of systematic reviews of randomised trials, the bedrock of neo-positivistic medicine in the twenty-first century.

Moreover, as society has become medicalised, the incidents of adverse reactions to medical intervention have increased exponentially. Drugs are swallowed by people everywhere on a daily basis, reasons Illich, so many will be injecting the wrong drug, or taking the wrong dosage. Some will be unwittingly concocting a lethal combination of chemicals formed from these drugs and food-stuffs containing artificial colouring or insecticides. Others, particularly those in the developing countries, will be given contaminated batches, and may also be vulnerable to secondary diseases from unsterilised needles used to inject the drugs into the body. A number (for example, the tens of millions who take tranquillisers) will become addicted to their medication.

Those who take antibiotics routinely will lower their resistance to future disease by altering the body's existing flora thereby becoming receptive to more resistant and mutating organisms. Virtually all of those on medication will suffer from one or multiple side-effects from a list of hundreds of thousands. These side-effects may be so severe as to be life threatening. Moreover, the overuse of antibiotics, both in humans and animals, is a huge threat to public health all across the globe. Strains of bacteria ('superbugs') have developed which are menace to whole populations, requiring new antibiotics to be formulated. For example, methycillin-resistant staphylococcus aureus (MRSA), a bacteria which cannot be killed by any conventional antibiotic, has spread throughout hospitals in Europe, North America and Japan. Vancomycin-intermediate staph aureus (VISA), a bacteria resistant to hitherto known antibiotics is also proliferating. Impregnable variations of tubercle-bacillus, malaria, gonorrhoea, meningitis and typhoid, which continue to kill tens of millions of people per year, are exported from infected areas to countries that had previously either never had the disease or from where it had been eradicated. Modern international transport systems and migration of great swathes of people from one geographical region to another, means that nowhere is safe from teratoid micro-organisms.

It has been estimated that in one year 20,000 people who died during surgery in Britain should not have had an operation in the first place (DoH 1998b). These patients died either because they were too frail to undertake an operation, particularly where a general anaesthetic was given, or due to faulty medical procedures (i.e. their operation was unnecessary, or they contracted post-operative infections which subsequently killed them). Furthermore, the incidents of 'law-suit laparotomies' are swelling in the USA, and will probably grow in Britain. That is, due to the litigious nature of the North American consumers, and the huge pay-outs made where medical negligence has been proven, doctors are asking for full investigations, including diagnostic surgery, to be made when patients complain of the most trivial of symptoms. Such excessive explorations are undertaken so that the doctor avoids being sued if a serious illness is uncovered at some later date.

Adverse drug reactions kill a further 20,000 people in Britain every year, and in the USA are reckoned to be the fourth highest cause of death (106,000 per annum) after heart disease, cancer and cerebro-vascular accidents (Dobson 1998). Lethal reactions to medication are, in the vast majority of cases, the result of the chemical make-up of the drug in question interfering with the functioning of organs (such as the damaging effect of paracetamol on the liver, or aspirin on the stomach), or the result of the patient not properly following the instructions on dosage. In other cases there is a catastrophic response by the body (anaphylaxis) to the drug which may produce immediate death. Up to 20 per cent of all hospital admissions are due to adverse drug reactions.

Cosmetic surgery is able to offer larger or smaller breasts, a reshaped nose, the sucking out or tucking in of adipose tissue, a lifted face, thicker lips and an enlarged penis. Advertising for such operations is prevalent within most popular magazines and newspapers. But the repugnant repercussions for some patients who have undergone such resectioning of their bodies are now realised. For example, breast implants made of such materials as silicone and soya can cause long-lasting health problems, and leave the patient in a worse condition (physically and emotionally) than she was prior to seeking help from the growing band of aesthetic surgeons.

In a magnificent example of 'iatrogenic-irony', the Consumers' Association (1999) in its independent review of drugs and therapeutics, reported that readily available painkilling tablets taken by people who suffer from chronic 'tension' headaches may be making their condition worse. That is, where an individual takes more than twelve doses per week, the severity of her or his symptoms would not be reversed, but would increase. If the painkiller was discontinued the original headache may be found to have gone, but pain as a result of taking the anti-headache medication would not necessarily stop!

Illich offers a 'radical utopian' solution to the disempowering effect of the professions. He predicts an eventual nemesis for the professions:

> Professional cartels are now as brittle as the French clergy in the age of Voltaire; soon, the still inchoate post-professional ethos will reveal the iron cage of their nakedness ... But unbeknownst

to them their credibility fades fast. A post-professional ethos takes shape in the spirit of those who begin to see the emperor's true physiognomy.

(see Illich in Illich *et al.* 1977: 37)

Illich advocates the de-professionalisation of all professions, together with the de-industrialisation of the developed world's economic base. Industrial society would be replaced by a system of 'intermediate' technology. He argues also for the retention and protection of craftwork. Technological production would be based on the needs of the community, rather than on the over-stimulated 'wants' created by gigantic and alienating industrial conglomerates – and the professionals.

The problem with the radical utopian approach, however, is that, apart from spontaneous revolution, there is little elucidation on how industrial society is to go through such a permutation. Nor is there qualification of exactly what is meant by 'intermediate' technology, or what mechanisms would be put in place to, on the one hand, prevent unacceptable growth, and on the other, ensure against technological decline (Richman 1987). Moreover, since the 1970s (when Illich began his crusade for smaller-scale and locally based economies), the economic agenda has altered spectacularly. Despite the existence of a number of experiments in 'intermediate technology' found in various parts of the world, supra-national economic developments, aided by global communication networks, have produced a 'universal market'. Industrialisation and capitalism have expanded rather than contracted. Furthermore, the former socialist countries in Eastern Europe, with their proclaimed needs-led economies, are attempting to respond to the industrial exigencies of capitalism. Communist China, facilitated by the reclaimed Hong Kong, is unashamedly industrialising on a massive scale.

More specifically, however, there is a need for a realistic approach to particular treatments that from Illich's perspective may be far too unsafe to be prescribed. Take the example of the acne drug Roaccutane, taken by nearly ten million people worldwide since its marketing in the early 1980s, that has been linked to suicide. Where suicide has allegedly occurred, there is no doubt that this is a devastating side-effect of a modern medicine. However, where acne is a physically disfiguring, psychologically damaging and chronic affliction, Roaccutane may be considered to be a tremendous boon to the quality of life of its users. This is especially so when many sufferers are in their teenage years, and already feel under pressure to be presentable to their peers and to prospective sexual partners. Moreover, having severe acne may not only force sufferers to retreat socially, but can conceivably be in itself a determinant of suicide. This is not to argue that the overall benefit of the drug is worth the risk of suicide. But doctors are expected to offer pills, potions and incisions to remedy distressing conditions, and may have to make decisions on the basis of the best of two evils – either let the patient endure her or his torment, or satisfy a requisition for succour and gamble that the cure will not be worse than the complaint.

Illich is suggesting that humans need to tolerate their afflictions, and that not to do so is reducing their appreciation of 'being' in the world. Those who succumb to the wares of the medical profession are somehow ontologically substandard. But the reality of pain and suffering from acne, cancer, childbirth, toothache, or depression, for most of us means that we perhaps are quite willing to give up an element of our ontological sovereignty to whoever wishes to administer relief and/or thwart an early death.

Healthism

The prevention of illness and maintenance of health has become a permeating standard by which many (if not all) behaviours (drinking, eating, work and leisure) are judged. This is what Crawford (1980), taking a lead from Zola (1977), has described as *healthism*. There has been an explosion of commercial and politically-sponsored interest in exercise, jogging, diets, vitamins, fitness machines and anti-stress measures. There is an aggressive anti-smoking, anti-alcohol ethic and a social stigma attached to perceptions of 'overeating'. There has also been a rise in the holistic health movement. These developments have resulted in the *medicalisation* of the normal rather than just the deviant, and form the thrust of contemporary health promotion policies by national governments and international agencies such as WHO. Self-care and healthy living are the predominant maxims of health service propaganda.

A day in the life of an erstwhile unreformed and unhealthy citizen consists of: a pre-breakfast cigarette, followed by a fried and high fat meal (eggs, sausages, 'black pudding', white bread, a hot beverage with full-cream milk and two spoonfuls of granulated sugar); a drive to work, where a sedentary role is performed, punctuated by serial caffeinated coffee consumption, and sporadic bouts of smoking (perhaps in a huddle with other health reprobates outside of the workplace building); an alcohol-rich lunch, with chips; chocolate and cake during break-times; a drive home via the public house for alcoholic refreshments; an evening of 'couch-potato' leisure pursuits with accompanying alcoholic refurbishment, and at least one high-calorie feast, with chips; and finally, a cigarette either prior to, or following, an unfulfilling sexual act and a night of fitful sleep.

A day in the life of a reconstituted health-conscious citizen consists of: pre-breakfast physical exertions, followed by cholesterol-reducing organic porridge, and high-fibre wholemeal bread; a jog to the place of employment; any food consumed at work consists only of (diet) soft drinks, de-caffeinated herbal tea, low-calorie biscuits; participation in the employer's mandatory exercise-breaks; an aerobic session at the health club on return from work; an evening meal of vegetarian *nouvelle cuisine*, two (small) glasses of (red) wine, and a multivitamin tablet with added minerals; and finally a soothing sexual encounter, and the reading of articles on self-improvement, preceding a restful night's sleep.

Healthy behaviour is reinforced by a myriad of 'fitness' images displayed in shops. Most of the magazines in the racks of newsagents project in visual and textual forms slim (women), muscular (men), and sexualised bodies and minds (both genders).

Failure to maintain health is regarded as a failure of will. Healthy behaviour becomes the model for 'good living', and healthy people are 'good/ideal' citizens. But, the promotion of 'autonomy' over one's life and health is in reality the promotion of oppression. Bodies and minds are regulated by the 'health police', an amalgam of medical practitioners, nurses and other paramedics, politicians and industrialists.

Healthism, from the constructionist viewpoint, is part of the 'consumerisation of everything' in society. Health has been procured as a commodity within a culture in which there is rampant commodification of all personal and social habits. For Roger Burrows and his co-theorists, *healthism* (signified by, for example, representations of youthfulness, vitality, energy, invigoration and sexiness) has become a core platform of post-modern culture:

In the 1960s a list of 'health-related' commodities would have
included such items as aspirins, TCP, Dettol and plasters. Today, however, it would include: food and drink [and] health
promoting pills; private health; alternative medicine; exercise
machines and videos; health insurance; membership of health
and sport clubs; walking boots; running shoes; cosmetic surgery; shampoo (for 'healthy looking hair'). ...

(Burrows *et al.* 1995: 2)

For Featherstone *et al.* (1991) a process of 'transvaluation' has
occurred. That is, the original function of and significance given to
goods or habits has altered to incorporate 'supra' or extra values
and meanings. For example, exercise is no longer merely for fun, but
an expression of a healthy lifestyle. Moreover, the accompanying
products in the playing of games such as football, tennis, squash or
badminton, all have logos or are styled in particular ways that
signify status rather than use.

It is not, however, just health that is being commodified, but the
body and its parts. For example, human eggs and sperm are
extracted and stored, to be used when the right 'customer' comes
along. Human reproductive cells are sold on the Internet. Those
that have been donated by models, whose photographs appear in the
cyber-advert, can command a price of up to $15,000 for one ovum
or dollop of sperm (Carter 1999).

Furthermore, there are moves allegedly by biotechnology companies to patent segments of the human genetic code for commercial reasons (Borger 1999). The unravelling of the human genetic
code offers the prospect of major medical advances, as well as
colossal profits if the rights to the knowledge of how genes work
are commandeered by capitalist enterprises. The blueprint to life
itself will then be for sale.

Summary

Society has become indoctrinated by medical and health concepts.
We focus on gaining health and avoiding disease to the detriment of
alternative ways of giving meaning to our lives. Not to be healthy,
or not employing strategies to obtain good health, attracts the tag
of 'deviant' and is considered to be socially reprehensible.

The 'health police' (whose ranks include nurses) are monitoring
more and more behaviours and an ever larger proportion of the

population. Health deviants (the fat, ugly, unfit, diseased, deformed and sexually unattractive) will be susceptible not only to increased levels of social disgrace, but could eventually face obligatory medical intervention or the withdrawal of health services.

Further reading

Illich, I. (1977) *Limits to Medicine – Medical Nemesis: The Expropriation of Health*, Harmondsworth: Penguin.

Chapter 7

Inequality

The social foundation of health and illness is stark and conspicuous when the issue of how incidents of serious diseases and early death affect the working class, poor and excluded. In Britain before the twentieth century the greatest killers, especially of children, were infectious diseases (for example, tuberculosis and diphtheria). From the 1920s onwards the biggest killers of adults became cancer, heart disease and cerebro-vascular accidents. All of these biological malefactions have been far more virulent amongst the underprivileged than the privileged.

Over a twenty-year period (1980–2000) the evidence amassed from study after study attests to an individual's position in the social hierarchy being a major determinant of morbidity and mortality. Therefore, inequalities in society (in terms of wealth, power, prestige and social inclusion/exclusion) are far more important factors in the maintenance of good health and the creation of disease than those that emerge from biology.

Moreover, these social disparities are replicated globally, with the health of the poorer nations far worse, and life expectancy far lower, than in richer parts of the world. Within Europe there are also extensive differences between the morbidity rates (especially levels of cardio-vascular disease) and the life expectancy of people living in the western part compared with those living in the central and eastern parts (Brunner and Marmot 1999). Furthermore, the divergence in health status between Russia and the countries in the west of Europe is particularly apparent. Russia has reversed its improved life expectancy since the days of the Soviet Union. This also seems to hold true for those countries that were formerly part of the Soviet Union. Rates of coronary heart disease amongst Swedish and Lithuanian men were cognate. But by 1994 (following the dissolution of the Soviet empire) death from coronary heart disease had quadrupled in Lithuania (Brunner and Marmot 1999).

There is, as the World Bank (1993) has recognised, an unmistakable link between the gross national product (GNP) of a country and the life expectancy of its population. An increase in the GNP of a poor country will result in an exponential rise in life expectancy.

In relative terms, the gap between marginalised and dominant groups within Western society is growing. The same is apparent between the developed (industrialised/post-industrialised) and the developing (industrialising) world. In this sense, therefore, the term 'developing' to describe those countries that are less commensurate than they were with the industrialised areas of the world is erroneous.

Difference in health provision and access can also be enormous between developed countries. The experience of British journalist Alan Wilkinson (1997) of becoming ill when visiting New York is illuminating. The USA with its largely private insurance system, supplies minimal 'free' provision in its public hospitals. Although carrying holiday insurance, he attends the local public hospital as he has difficulty in breathing, and is (eventually) diagnosed as having pneumonia. Apart from the not unexpected wait in a crowded casualty department for four hours, and the highly predictable indignity of being asked what language the English speak by the registration attendant, he found that he was the only white patient. A further extensive wait of five hours for a bed gave him the opportunity to observe closely his fellow patients and the actions of the medical staff:

> There was a junkie, collapsed across two chairs. There was the woman with the blood-soaked leg. 'That mother-f*****! I shoulda killed him', she groaned. There was the hero on crutches, grimacing manfully. 'Hey, it's where the bullet lodged, man. Kinda pus and blood oozing out, right?'. And then there was the demented, neglected, rotting poor. A Hispanic woman wrapped in a bathrobe. 'Ees my legs doctor'. He gestured with his stethoscope. There were no concessions to modesty. Just 'Open Up'. ... A morose Nicaraguan peeled off a sock to reveal a rotten foot almost split in two. The doctor asked a colleague if he thought it was safe to touch it. The consensus was he'd better not: give the guy a jar of Vitamin E jelly and get him out.
>
> (Wilkinson 1997)

To tackle disease and premature death effectively, inequalities have to be addressed, which may demand major 'cultural' changes in the way in which people conduct their lives, the internal structure of society, and in the economic relations between first- and third-world countries. Therein lies the problem. Although ostensibly there is at times the political will by governments to grapple with inequality nationally and internationally, little would seem to have been achieved.

Moreover, in Britain the National Health Service (NHS), set up in 1946 with the explicit mandate of harmonising the health status of people at the lower end of the social scale with that found among people at the top, has not been successful. Overall, the health of all groups in society has improved, but nearly sixty years of medical (and nursing) interventions within the framework of the NHS appears to have had the paradoxical effect of making people further down the social hierarchy comparatively more sick.

Black Report

In 1977 the Working Group on Inequalities in Health, chaired by Sir Douglas Black, the former Chief Scientist at the Department of Health, was commissioned by the then Labour government. The terms of reference for the working group were:

1   to bring together available information about the differences in health status among the social classes, and about contributing factors;
2   to analyse the collected information for causal relationships;
3   to assess the implication for health and social policy, and to suggest in what direction further research should be taken.

Three years later, in 1980 the working group produced its findings (known as the Black Report: Townsend *et al.* 1992), and presented these to the Tory government of Margaret Thatcher which had won the 1979 election. The new government, however, treated the report with indifference and then disdain. A mere few hundred copies were made available by the Department of Health; no press conference was called; and only a limited number of journalists were informed of the report. Moreover, the press agencies were sent information about the report on the Friday prior to a public holiday weekend, thereby attracting very little publicity even where journalists took the trouble to report its findings.

However, an 'unofficial' meeting with the press was held at the Royal College of Physicians. The media attention that followed prompted a reaction from the Secretary of State for Health, who disowned the report, claiming that the enormous cost of implementing its advice (calculated at the time to be in excess of £2 billion) was prohibitive.

The working party had concluded that at all stages of life, people belonging to the lower social classes (as measured by the Registrar General's hierarchy of occupational groups), had a comparatively worse health experience. Taking the two-year period of 1970 to 1972, the Black Report disclosed that 74,000 more lives had been lost from the semi-skilled and unskilled occupational groups than from the top (professional) group. Ten thousand of the dead had been children.

The specific observations of the Black Report were:

1   There are marked differences in mortality rates between the occupational groups, for both sexes, and in all age groups.
2   Twice as many babies born to unskilled manual parents (Registrar General's group V) die within the first month of life compared to babies born to parents in the professional occupational class (Registrar General's group I).
3   Approximately three times as many infants born to unskilled manual parents die within the first year of life compared to babies born to parents in the professional occupational class. Rates of self-reported chronic illness are twice as high among men in the unskilled occupational class compared to men in the professional occupational class.
4   Rates of self-reported chronic illness are two and a half times as high amongst wives of men in the unskilled occupational class compared to wives of men in the professional occupational class.
5   Men and women from the unskilled manual occupational class are two and a half times more likely to die before reaching the age of retirement compared to men and women in the professional occupational class.

Significantly, however, the Black Report gave notification that the health system itself could not in any dramatic way alter these figures. The key social (rather than health) issues were – and still are – unemployment, lack of decent education, shoddy housing and inadequate transport to connect people with essential services such as shops and medical facilities. The tenor of the thirty-seven recommendations made in the Black Report was that, in order to reduce health inequalities, there had to be a major increase in public expenditure to improve working and living conditions. That is, the structure of society needs to be altered. '*In our view much of the evidence on social inequalities in health can be adequately understood in terms of specific features of the socio-economic environment*' (Black Report in Townsend *et al.* 1992: 199, emphases in the original).

There are other explanations for inequalities in health, however, besides that which views the organisation of society and material conditions setting the scene for an individual's lifestyle. From the interactionist perspective people make meaningful choices about how to conduct their lives. For example the decision to smoke, indulge in heavy drinking, take little physical exercise and eat high-fat foods, is not the result of active coercion by the owners of the industries selling these products, their advertising agents or 'free-market' politicians. Moreover, the individual's micro- and macro-cultural affiliations and interactions may be sufficiently cogent to reduce the effects of structural pressures. Through daily interaction with friends, family, working colleagues and the surrounding community, the individual is likely to have her or his behaviour modified. It is far easier to maintain a healthy eating and exercise regime if one's partner, peers and business associates are like-minded. Equally, if an individual's interactions are with groups that have norms associated with drugs and lethargy, then the chances are that she or he will follow suit.

The 'social selection' perspective advances a variation of Darwin's theory of natural section (West 1991). That is, social class is viewed as the outcome of an involuntary and evolutionarily determined sorting process that is 'normal' for human populations. It is argued from this paradigm that some people are genetically more physically and mentally capable than others, and this will inevitably result in a rank order based on how fit a person is in the race to survive. These innate physical and psychological characteristics mean that some individuals are born to have bad health and to die early, and the same group will be social underachievers. Hence, the low occupational classes contain most of the unhealthy people in society not because of any causal relationship between the two, as is propounded by both the structuralists and the interactionists, but because they 'naturally' occur together. Those with physical and mental health problems will 'drift' into the disadvantaged strata of society as a matter of course. The physically and mentally advantaged will maintain good health and gain social superiority. Self-evidently, unemployed people are more likely to be ill than are people with successful careers, and also the reverse is true.

However, Margaret Whitehead (in Townsend *et al.* 1992) examines the evidence, and argues that inter-generational social mobility is far more dependent on educational, cultural and material factors than health. That is, illness does not in the main cause a downward spiral of social mobility. Notwithstanding any illness present, it is much more probable that where a family values educational attainment and is financially assured, any progeny will either be as successful as the parents, or be propelled into a higher class. As far as intra-generational movement is concerned, if serious illness occurs in childhood then this can affect social mobility. Long-term conditions such as respiratory disease and schizophrenia, if contracted at an early age, may produce a drift down the social scale, but the number affected in this way only accounts for a small proportion of those who are ill and indigent.

Furthermore, whilst organic and evolutionary drives may play their part in shaping behaviour, these would not logically be pushing the individual in the direction of self-destruction. That is, swallowing large numbers of hamburgers, drinking copious amounts of intoxicating beverages, inhaling habitually noxious substances and avoiding any physical exertion beyond walking to the public house or tobacconist, are not compatible with biological survival. Whatever bio-genetic imperatives there are in human behaviour, these are patently overridden by the effects of cultural interactions and social structures with respect to health inequalities.

What the contributors to the Black Report made clear was that the greatest contributory factor to variations in health was social inequality. In particular, the Black Report advocated (1) a movement away from a 'disease-based' health system towards prevention, and community and primary services; (2) a radical improvement in the material conditions of vulnerable groups, particularly children and the disabled, both in terms of financial support, housing and employment.

Tory ministers at the time countered that the recommendations of the Black Report were too expensive for any government to install (arguing that the total cost had already risen to nearly £5 billion a year after the publication of the report). The Tory government also claimed that research other than that covered in the report led to different conclusions about the cause of ill health amongst the poor. Townsend *et al.* (1992) suggest that the financial argument against interfering with social inequalities to improve health is faulty. Merely using the raw figure of how expensive the recommendations of the Black Report would be to implement ignores the hidden social and economic cost of health inequalities. By allowing people to die too young, suffer serious illness and work in hazardous conditions, society is not only losing out in terms of productivity but is heading towards moral bankruptcy. They posit that expenditure on armaments could be diverted into health.

However, the structuralist perspective has been contested from a different stance to that taken by either the interactionists or the evolutionary theorists. The 'artefact' approach not only attacks the way in which research about health inequalities has been conducted, but by inference assails much of what purports to be social-scientific thought (Illsley 1986).

From the artefact position, sociology is accused of 'inventing' concepts to explain phenomena that may not exist in the first instance. That is, when sociologists refer to 'social structure', 'inequality', 'poverty' and 'social exclusion', they are formulating ideas about what is real in the world that either have little validity or may be based on false assumptions. From this point of view, social scientists merely select certain 'facts' and formulate abstract notions about their significance. Moreover, from this insecure epistemological basis, presumptions are made about the correlation these facts have with other facts. For example, the continued occurrence of health inequalities may not have any direct relationship to the material situation of the group at the bottom of the social hierarchy – particularly as there has been a three-fold rise in the value of average incomes since the beginning of the 1970s. Indeed, the gap in health status between the groups can be viewed as spurious as the bottom group has shrunk as a proportion of the population. Consequently, there are in both absolute and relative numbers far fewer chronically ill people and early deaths arising from this social stratum.

Moreover, the placing of people into occupational class categories is an artificial process. The formulation of a series of groups on the premise of the status of a person's employment is based on certain subjective judgements. For example, a lawyer (occupational group I) may earn much more than a plumber (occupational group III). But the latter may be more content with her or his life, and if self-employed, have a much greater level of freedom at work, and more opportunities for leisure compared to an employee of a busy law practice.

The situation is complicated somewhat by the position taken by extreme constructionist sociologists who also perceive all social and natural phenomena to be fabricated. Therefore, some sociologists are contributing to the artefact case by implying that such diseases as cancer and coronary infarction cannot be taken as given, let alone the social identity of those believed to be more prone to contracting these conditions.

Furthermore, the comparison over long periods of time, of the health of any group of workers is likely to be misleading. The role performance of manual workers today, in what is left of the manufacturing industry, is governed by very different rules and expectations, and health and safety regulations, to that which could be found in the factories and mines at the start of the twentieth century. As Peter Aggleton cautions: 'It is vitally important, therefore, to be aware of the limitations of the categories used to classify data in health research' (Aggleton 1990: 27).

Whitehead (in Townsend *et al.* 1992) points out, however, that a mass of evidence has indicated that there are actual differences in health between social groups, and these cannot be dismissed as statistical blips. Longitudinal studies, projects that have controlled for trends in employment over time, and research that has used indicators of social status other than occupational class, do not alter in any great detail the conclusions reached in the Black Report.

One classic longitudinal piece of research that deserves special mention in the debate about the relevance of the structuralist perspective is the 'Whitehall Study'. Michael Marmot and his colleagues (Marmot *et al.* 1984) carried out an analysis of the health of 17,000 male civil servants based in London over many years, starting at the end of the 1960s. At the beginning of the study the civil servants were examined medically to provide a baseline of their health. After seven years, more than 1,000 had died, with the cause of death myocardial infarction in half of the cases. However, there were higher death rates amongst the lower grades of workers compared to those with senior positions, with the death-rate gradient being proportionate to each tier of seniority. The lower grades of civil servants had almost four times the death rate of the very top civil servants.

What is important here is that the organisational hierarchy corresponded to the health–disease status of the employees. Evidence from this study, therefore, implies that relative deprivation rather than absolute deprivation is the significant determinant of morbidity and mortality. Furthermore, even where no detectable disease was discernible at the start of the study, the lower the grade the higher the death rate. That is, any recruitment of diseased civil servants to work in unskilled roles could not account for the mortality rate in this group.

Hence, Marmot *et al.* (1984) demonstrated that occupational status is a robust predictor of such life-threatening conditions as coronary heart disease. Coronary heart disease is one of the biggest causes of death in England, with 115,000 people dying each year (DoH 1999b).

Moreover, they argued that employment grades were actually more indicative of coronary disease than smoking, high cholesterol and hypertension. To test out this proposition more fully, a second study of civil servants was embarked upon using a sample of 4,691 men and 1,903 women (Marmot *et al.* 1991). Biological (for example, carbohydrate metabolism and rates of blood clotting) and somatic (for example, abdominal fat levels) indicators of the potential to suffer from coronary disease and diabetes were found to be associated with employees in lower-grade positions. Once again, there was a correlation between (in this case future) ill-health and the relative occupational status. Moreover, certain work-based psycho-social factors such as how much autonomy and variety or direction and monotony were experienced by employees, appeared to be critical. An insight from the study was that both men and women in lower civil-service grades reported that they had less control over their work, were given repetitive and unskilled tasks and had a slower pace of work, compared with those in higher grades, and that job satisfaction was correspondingly lower.

Absence from work because of sickness was coupled to occupational grade and perceptions of job satisfaction. Whether measuring short periods of absence (i.e. under seven days) or longer terms (seven days or over), dissatisfied lower-grade employees were much more likely to be off work. The most unhappy employees in the lowest ranks had up to six times the rate of sickness of the highest-ranking and content employees.

The policies that were given support by the Tory government following the publication of the Black Report were based on health education programmes, personal responsibility and the use of the voluntary sector in health and social services. Whilst it is true that succeeding Tory governments recognised the structural background to health inequalities, there still remained an overriding emphasis on individual culpability and control compared to that indicated in the research presented in the Black Report.

This was most certainly the case in *The Health of the Nation*, launched in the early 1990s (DoH 1992). This document reinforced the individual as the locus of change. At the heart of the approach was the notion that information about healthy lifestyles should be disseminated effectively so that people could make their own decisions about what to eat, how much exercise to indulge in and what medical services should be used or bought. It has had long-term influence over health promotion programmes, which remain predicated on the empowerment of people to make 'healthier choices'. As Jenny Douglas (1996) comments, the health of the nation policy did not incorporate within its philosophy a realisation that many people are constrained in their ability to make healthy choices by the social, economic and political milieux in which they conduct their lives.

The link between social disparity and health inequality, due to the weight of evidence, is now taken more or less as 'proven' by both social scientists and policy makers. But there has not been a commitment by any subsequent government to provide the financial support for all of the prescriptions of the Black Report.

Health divide

As a follow-up to the Black Report, in 1987 the Health Education Council, shortly before its demise, published its report, 'The Health Divide' to much the same media and political furore. The evidence reviewed in this report (and in the updated version: Whitehead 1992), confirmed that serious inequalities in health had persisted throughout the 1980s and into the 1990s.

The notion of equity and fairness is central to the HEC report. There is, for example, an identification of the individual's right to reach her or his 'full health potential', or at least not be so disadvantaged that this prospect is unattainable. That is, governments should strive to ensure that as far as is possible the socio-economic climate engenders good health. Moreover, there should be access to care and treatment on the basis of need rather than on what standard of service happens to exist in a particular location, how much an individual can afford to pay, or to what social class, ethnic group, age category or gender that person belongs.

Whether measured by occupational class, by assets such as car and home ownership, or by employment status, a similar picture of health and illness had emerged, it was argued in 'The Health Divide'. People lower down the social scale died younger than those at the top of the scale. The inequality divide was increasing in all but one area of health. There had been dramatic headway made in the survival rates of babies aged one month to one year from every social group, and the infant mortality gap between the groups had narrowed considerably. However, babies born in the less-favoured occupational classes had a lower birth weight, and would tend to be shorter in height than their better-off peers.

As had been found by the researchers involved in the Black Report, semi-skilled and unskilled manual workers made less use of the preventative health services than the professional and quasi-professional groups. Axiomatically, the former groups had higher attendance rates for 'curative' interventions in general practitioners' surgeries.

The unemployed and their families were found to have considerably worse physical health than those in employment. A range of studies had concluded that unemployment causes a chronic deterioration in mental health which improves when those affected return to work. Whilst there is a marked difference in health trends between women and men (women having higher rates of sickness than men, but lower mortality rates), working-class women have noticeably poorer health than the better-off members of their gender.

The health profile of ethnic minority groups born outside of Britain, as one could expect given the dissimilar historical and cultural backgrounds to both the white majority and each other, is not straightforward. For example, Afro-Caribbean people have a much higher incidence of hypertension and cerebro-vascular disease than the British average for all groups, and people of Asian extraction are more susceptible to heart disease.

Crucially, the HEC found that the number of children living in privation had increased, demonstrating that family welfare policies in this area had failed. Moreover, welfare benefits had been ineffectual with regard to nutrition, housing and protection from unsafe and unhealthy working practices.

A geographical split in Britain was also detected, which in the main follows a north-south cleavage. Death rates were highest in Scotland, the north of England, and lowest in south-east England and East Anglia. However, as had been illustrated in a study by Townsend *et al.* (1987), of material deprivation and its effect on health in the zone covered by the Northern Regional Health Authority, there are huge variations within communities. That is, many localities have sub-districts that contain populations with very poor health and living in sub-standard material circumstances, alongside sub-districts with much better health and social conditions.

In conclusion, the HEC report was forthright in its advocacy of material change in society, suggesting four broad strategies:

> ensuring an adequate income for all; improving living condi-
> tions and the chance to obtain housing in the first place; im-
> proving working conditions and the chance of safe and
> fulfilling employment; and removing barriers to the adoption of
> healthy personal lifestyles.
>
> (Whitehead 1992: 393)

The HEC argued that there had never been a nationally co-ordinated plan on equalities in health. Therefore, these strategies could form such a plan, but to be effective would need the combined involvement and goodwill of local social and health authorities and relevant government departments.

Healthier nation

Margaret Whitehead had hoped when she wrote the preface to the second edition of 'The Health Divide' (1992) that, as health inequalities worsened in Britain and in countries such as Sweden and the Netherlands (both of which had previously been renowned for equality in health provision), they would be taken much more seriously. That is, as the health of the socially segregated worsened throughout Europe, the press, public and politicians would no longer be able to avoid the stark reality of this group's plight. Homelessness amongst the young, and lack of resources in the community for the mentally disordered, would become too obvious to ignore as these people could be seen to be in distress on the streets of British cities. The expanding gap between the healthy and the diseased would reach such an outrageous level, with perhaps decades separating the lifespan of the rich from the poor, that a much more pro-active attempt to tackle structural inequalities would have to be considered.

When the New Labour government was elected in 1997 explicit recognition of the interconnection of health and social disparities was voiced. The then Secretary of State for Health, Frank Dobson, was forthright in his portrayal of the health–poverty connection and the willingness of New Labour politicians to carry out an effective strategy to ameliorate the situation they had inherited from the Tories:

> The whole programme of the Government amounts to a cru-
> sade against health inequalities. ... Every Government Depart-
> ment is joined up and signed up to tackle the things that make
> people ill – poverty, low pay, unemployment, poor housing,
> environmental pollution, crime and disorder. It's a fact that
> poor people are ill more often and die sooner. Over the last two
> decades the gap between rich and poor people has grown. The
> gap between rich and poor neighbourhoods has grown. ... So
> we are targeting help on the families and areas that have suf-
> fered most deprivation and most ill health.
>
> (Dobson quoted in DoH 1998a: 1)

Two years later, there were manifest commitments to structural transformations. In the White Paper *Saving Lives: Our Healthier Nation* (DoH 1999b), the New Labour government gave support to the structuralist position by acknowledging that the factors which harm people's health, such as air pollution, unemployment, low wages and poor housing, are beyond the control of any single individual.

The second post-1997 Secretary of State for Health of the New Labour government (appointed in 1999 to replace Frank Dobson) was equally unambiguous in recognising the relationship between social inequality and ill-health. Referring specifically to the unequal distribution of heart disease in Britain, in a commentary published on the front page of a national broadsheet newspaper, Alan Milburn connects the two political soundbites of 'healthier nation' and 'fairer nation':

> Although heart disease claims more than 140,000 deaths a year in Britain, its effects are distributed unequally: the death rate amongst skilled men is almost three times higher than among professionals. In the past two decades the differences in mortality have more than doubled. These stark facts spell out why tackling heart disease is one of the keys not only to a healthier nation but to a fairer nation too.
>
> (Milburn 1999)

Milburn also admits to the existence of inequality in access to specialist cardiac services. That is, in the parts of Britain where the rate of heart disease is high there are fewer expert cardiac surgeons employed and therefore less surgical interventions carried out.

Having accepted the proposition that socio-economic elements have to be addressed in order to harvest a healthier nation, there is a covenant given by the government to take action. That is, within the document is a commitment to some form of social change. Specifically, many of the post-1997 New Labour government's policies were designed to alter the material position of those in poverty, and to help the socially excluded re-engage with mainstream society. For example, unemployment was addressed by the 'New Deal'. This entailed encouraging employers to offer 'extra' (low-paid) jobs through the use of financial subsidies to people such as unqualified school-leavers who might otherwise remain chronically unemployed. This government also introduced a national minimum wage, aimed at helping the very worst-paid employees. Furthermore, strategies aimed at reducing pollutants from motor vehicles, and improving the housing stock were embarked upon.

However, by no means was this a fully fledged materialist doctrine in operation. There was to be no social revolution, or forced and cogent redistribution of wealth, but the installation of 'health action zones', 'healthy living centres' and improved medical provision. Moreover, the New Labour government made no guarantee of short- or even medium-term solutions, with the Secretary of State for

Health openly acknowledging that 'we [the government] have a long way to go' (Milburn 1999) to provide a healthier and fairer nation. Whilst social, economic and environmental ingredients are recognised as 'potent' in the creation of disease, the Blairite 'Third Way' is conferred to health care in the shape of combining the government's structural obligations with that of individual responsibility.

That is, there is explicit reference to the control an individual has in making decisions about her or his lifestyle, and about the health needs of the family. For example, a family may be poor, live in a terrible dwelling in the shadow of a noxious industrial plant or motorway, but mum and dad still can determine whether or not their children eat fruit and vegetables as opposed to chocolate and chips. The example of smoking is given in *Saving Lives: Our Healthier Nation* (DoH 1999b) to indicate how people do have the obligation to themselves and others to resist habits that are extremely damaging to health. One in four people will die from cancer, and this disease kills 127,000 people each year. A third of all cancer deaths are related to smoking.

However, smoking is the *cause célèbre* in the political and personal jurisdiction over health. The lighted cigarette epitomises the struggle an impoverished individual may have in governing her or his life. From the perspective of individual volition, inhaling tobacco is either the last act of wilful resistance to the daily grind of life by members of the underclass, or an incredible and asinine feat of self-destruction. From the perspective of social determinism, smoking signifies the predestined outcome of repressive forces in society. Moreover, whilst governments remonstrate with smokers about the dangers of tobacco, and ban cigarette advertising, the industries that manufacture these hazardous products are free to make profits and pay taxes.

Two years into the New Labour government's first term of office, the annual report of the New Policy Institute, *Monitoring Poverty and Social Exclusion* (Howarth et al. 1999) pointed out that there is no general pattern of improvement in poverty and inequality. Health inequalities continue to expand, with premature deaths becoming more geographically concentrated in poor areas. Incidents of obesity now occur almost three times more frequently amongst the Registrar General's social classes IV and V compared with social class I. Babies born into social classes IV and V have a 20 per cent greater chance of being underweight compared with those born into social classes I, II and III. The number of accidental deaths is falling but children in social classes IV and V are more than twice as likely to die in this way than children in social classes I, II and III.

Moreover, the report *The Widening Gap* argues that the actions of the New Labour government are not leading to a reversal of social and health inequalities, and that the life expectancy gap between social class I and men in social class V is 9.5 years for men and 6.4. for women (Shaw *et al.* 1999). In the report, attention is paid in particular to the geographical (or 'spatial') disparities in health throughout the country, contrasting all of the parliamentary constituencies. The evidence indicates that the death rates for 'worst health' constituencies are over two and a half times that of the 'best health' constituencies. Infant mortality is twice as likely in the 'worst health' constituencies compared to the 'best health' constituencies. For the authors of this report the simple fact is that twenty years after the Black Report, and thirteen years after 'The Health Divide':

> at the very end of the 20th century inequalities in health are extremely wide and are still widening in Britain. These inequalities are shown most clearly through the premature deaths of hundreds of thousands of people living in this country in the last two decades. We argue that such inequalities are patently unfair and that inequalities in health are the direct consequence of inequalities in wealth and the growth of poverty in Britain.
>
> (Shaw *et al.* 1999: 1)

For Richard Wilkinson (1999) the solution to health inequalities lies in attacking the structural determinants of the social environment. However, he does not believe that this means that economic growth should be relied on to provide better circumstances for the poor in the developed countries and for people in the developing parts of the world. He points out that improved economic performance may have a 'trickle-down' effect on social disadvantage. That is, those at the bottom of the social hierarchy benefit from the conspicuous consumption of those at the top due to, for example, the consequential increased employment. However, this, suggests Wilkinson, will only serve to re-enforce the differences in material wealth and health between social groups.

Wilkinson argues that the overall burden on society and the developing world of disadvantage needs to be addressed through the implementation of policies on employment, income and education. These policies must be aimed at altering the structural conditions that in turn foment social determinants of ill-health and premature death. He speculates that it is specifically income inequality which leads to a loss of a sense of dignity, self-respect and confidence. This then results in the atrophication of social relationships, which reduces further the individual's ability to cope with everyday life events. It is plausible, suggests Wilkinson, that these feeling of inferiority will induce chronic stress and thereby make the individual far more prone to infectious and cardiovascular diseases than if she or he felt valued by society.

This model, posits Wilkinson, helps to account for the concurrence of low social status, fragile or non-existent social networks, chronic anxiety and serious ill-health. Moreover, prolonged exposure to personal and social difficulties will exacerbate biological predilection to ill-health:

> A person's past social experiences become written into the physiology and pathology of their body. The social is, literally, embodied; and the body records the past, whether as an ex-officer's duelling scars or an ex-miner's emphysema. The duelling scar as a mark of social distinction, in turn predisposes to future advancement and social advantage, while the emphysema robs the employee of their labour and power and predisposes to future deprivation and social disadvantage.
>
> (Blane 1999: 64)

Wilkinson provides an example of the inadequacy of the 'individualistic' approach to health inequalities. He observes that there is already a public awareness of the health risks associated with inadequate and unwholesome diet, and inactivity. Political endeavour needs therefore not to be directed any more at the individual to eat healthily and jog more frequently, but at those food manufacturers who promote fatty beefburgers and highly sweetened drinks to children and salt-ridden, processed, ready meals to adults.

Moreover, the cost of healthy food is usually more than that of unhealthy food. Consequently, a remedy could be for government to install fiscal incentives that would redress this imbalance and enable those families on low wages or who are unemployed to make their choice of diet go beyond the consumption of cheap calories. As Wilkinson notes, foods and drinks soaked in sugar, fat and salt may be eaten 'for comfort' when people do not have lifestyle alternatives due to their material circumstances, and lack of educational and employment scope. Comfort foods, alcohol and smoking, provide a temporary escape from social oppression and personal despondency.

Summary

There is little doubt amongst social scientists (and even politicians) that there is an immutable conjunction between social inequalities and health inequalities. The evidence establishing the correlation between how healthy a person is and her or his social position began to be collected systematically at the end of the 1970s and continues to be amassed. The corollary of the appreciation of the effects of social structure on health is that the way in which society is organised must be modified – if not radically transformed – before the nation can be healthier. The work of nurses, doctors and other health-care practitioners without a political dimension based on this insight may be ineffectual if not counterproductive.

There is little sign of social reform on this scale being contemplated by politicians. The 2000 *National Health Service Plan* (DoH 2000a) will focus on increasing expenditure on health; reformulating doctors' contracts to reduce their involvement with private practice; improving patients' choice over treatment; levelling out provision to check the 'post-code lottery' of treatment being dependent upon where a patient lives; shortening waiting lists; and ensuring that hospitals are clean. It is a mandate for a shake-up of the NHS, not society.

Further reading

Shaw, M., Dorling, D., Gordon, D. and Smith, G.D. (1999) *The Widening Gap*, Bristol: Policy Press.

Chapter 8

Sex

Nurses are associated inescapably with sex. First, there are the sexual stereotypes. Female nurses are portrayed if not as virgin angels, then as sexual libertarians, libidinous, busty and adorned with starched aprons, black stockings and suspenders, and a coy manner. Alternative images present them as sexual prudes in the role of the middle-aged, overweight, domineering and repressed 'matron' figure. Male nurses are stereotyped as effeminate, homosexual, sexually incontinent, camp and in the wrong job because only female biology is thought to be capable of proliferating caring.

However, even though sexual connotations abound, nurses have perennially avoided the sexuality of their patients. At best lip-service has been paid to the sexual needs of those people who have been hospitalised, who are physically disabled, mentally disordered, suffer from learning difficulties, or are elderly. Illness disrupts sexuality. Health-care professionals customarily evade the question of how to compensate for the fundamental need for sexual expression. No matter how much attention is paid to 'holistic' nursing or medicine, this is one of the aspects of the patient's biological, psychological, social and spiritual needs spectrum that is neglected.

Second, nurses have a prime responsibility in the prevention and treatment of sexually transmitted disease. Sexual disease kills millions of people throughout the world. But sexual behaviour is tied to social practices. Therefore, to promote sexual health and prevent death by sex, knowledge of sexual pathology must be complemented by an understanding of the social context of human sexuality. Moreover, the promotion of sexual health goes beyond dealing with disease. Western governments and international health agencies are intent on encouraging people to be pro-active in obtaining the maximum quality in all areas of their lives. This includes being able to enjoy sex without unwanted consequences such as pregnancy. To be sexually healthy, therefore, is not just about the avoidance of disease but about reaching (or attempting to arrive at) the full potential of sexual experience.

Sexuality

Human sexuality, the gratification of carnal desire and/or the process by which the species is reproduced, is dynamic, elaborate, mostly pleasurable and potentially very dangerous. It is dynamic because it appears to drive a considerable amount of human behaviour, and operates on innumerable levels. Sex for humans is not just about creating babies, it can also bring immense enjoyment and satisfaction – if indulged in willingly, without abuse and with some degree of skill – either in order to procreate, or as an event in its own right. Sex, however, is risky. Unwanted babies, infection and untimely death are possible negative consequences of sexual congress.

At the biological level, sexual urges can be simply about the attraction that exists between men and women which leads to the 'mechanical' fertilisation of the female ovum by the male sperm. Heterosexual intercourse, the insertion of the man's erect penis into the woman's vagina, and the reaching of orgasm by the man, is the biological mechanism through which the woman can become pregnant. However, even this apparent uni-dimensional biological operation is very complex involving an interplay of many factors such as evolutionary pressures and the generation of sexually related bio-chemicals.

For the biologist, secretions from the pituitary gland following puberty stimulate the release of greater quantities of specific hormones (in men, testosterone, in women oestrogen and progesterone), and produce physiological changes. For men there is an increase in body hair, growth of muscle tissue (arms, legs, chest), lowering of the voice, enlargement of the penis and scrotum). For women there is the enlargement of the breasts, the growth of pubic and auxiliary hair, the reshaping of the contours of the body (shoulders, hips, buttocks, thighs) through the deposition of fat, the broadening of the pelvis, alterations to the linings of the uterus and vagina, and the commencement of menstruation. Whilst interest in certain aspects of sexuality is conceivable throughout infancy and childhood (for example, a small baby may gain sensual feelings from caressing her or his own genitals), fascination with sex is generally unabated amongst post-puberty adolescents.

However, evolutionary theorists argue that human sexuality, particularly the difference between male and female sexual behaviour, can be explained in terms of the species' 'reproductive strategy' that goes beyond the release of hormones at puberty. Humans have evolved a way of ensuring that offspring have the best chance of surviving. This involves men having sex with as many females as possible, whereas women have a tendency towards mating with only one male. Male promiscuity and female sexual conservatism is designed, argue the evolutionists, to allow the man to maximise his potential to reproduce his genes through disseminating liberally millions of spermatozoa, whereas the woman has to conserve her resources and protect her genetic investment given that she can only reproduce once every nine months. Thus, male licentiousness and capacity to carry out rape, and female sexual inertia and emotionalism, are reckoned to be integral to the process of successful procreation and the perpetuation of their respective genes.

Charles Darwin (1998, original 1859) presented the view that animals (and by implication therefore humans) were far more interested, in an evolutionary sense, in sex than survival. That is, animals would put themselves at risk from predators in order to attract a mate with whom to procreate. The passing on of genes was more important than continuation of the life of that animal.

For example, male frogs latch on to females for hours if not days during mating (thereby ensuring that no other male fertilises the female). This puts both in great danger from agile carnivores as the conjoint amphibians are restricted in their movements and cannot escape as easily as when they are not engaged in copulation. Thus the production of spawn becomes more pressing than escaping being swallowed by a snake.

There are, for Darwin, a number of essential components to sexual selection in animals that have application to humans. Male animals compete with other males for sex. This competition is won as a result of the greater physical strength, weaponry and attractiveness (additionally in the case of humans, intellectual power, social status and available resources such as property and money) of the victor.

> [Sexual selection] depends, not on a struggle for existence, but on a struggle between the males for possession of the females; the result is not death to the unsuccessful competitor, but few or no offspring. Sexual selection is, therefore, less rigorous than natural selection. Generally, the most vigorous males, those that are best fitted for their places in nature, will leave most progeny. But in many cases, victory depends not on general vigour, but on having special weapons, confined to the male sex. A hornless stag or spurless cock would have a poor chance of leaving offspring.
>
> (Darwin 1998, original 1859: 73)

The female is pro-active in the selection process by making preferences about a mate, and the male (to some extent) is responding to her demands. The qualities of the preferred mate re-emerge in subsequent generations of the species, whereas the attributes of the loser are destined to become extinct. It is she who is deciding about the best stag or cock.

Neo-evolutionary theorists such as David Buss (1994) have taken Darwin's elementary concept of sexual selection and attempted to refine and apply it to human mating behaviour. In a multi-staged study lasting five years and involving fifty collaborators, over 10,000 people from thirty-seven different cultures across the globe, aged between fourteen and seventy, Buss reports that much of what he found disturbed him. What his respondents registered was a 'ruthless pursuit of sexual goals'. Mates are not chosen at random. That is, from this research humans appear as strategists. They humiliate and denigrate rivals, deceive and manipulate possible mates, and subvert their actual mates, in order to achieve their sexual goals. For the evolutionist such apparently genuine and virtuous elements of human psychology as romance, love and caring, as well as nefarious dispositions such as jealousy, rage and emotional blackmail, contribute to the furthering of sexual objectives.

Conscious and unconscious mechanisms, allowing humans to adapt to all aspects of the physical and social environment, have ripened over millions of years. According to Buss, today's humans have inherited the aspirations of our ancestors. In the days of hunters and gatherers, what a female required was a mate who could protect her during the long and vulnerable period of pregnancy and child-rearing. She needed a successful supplier of food and heat, and a fighter to defend her from other males and dangerous animals. Therefore, women then, as today, desired men who could provide a stable and secure 'nest', and who could be counted on to be committed to a relationship and the offspring of that relationship. In Buss' study, women throughout the world and across ethnic and religious groups, and in all social classes, expressed a wish for financial collateral in a marriageable man. The trend by women to seek financial security was approximately double that sought by men. A powerful indication of economic viability in what women view as 'eligible men' is their high social status, or the likelihood (because of insinuated intelligence and ambition) of reaching an elevated position in society. Women wish to marry 'up' the social ladder, whereas men are much less choosy. Good physique remains on the sexual wish list for women tens of thousands of years after a large and muscular gladiator was needed to defend her from roaming sabre-toothed tigers and from being molested by (undesirable) men.

For men, youth is attractive in prospective mates as this is a patent declaration of reproductive capacity. Health, another fundamental reproductive requirement in women for men, is indicated by, for example, universally recognised notions of beauty. Although the significance of a woman's weight varies cross-culturally, a standard waist-to-hip ration of 0.7 or below gives the impression to the perusing male eye that the target of his sexual inspection is not pregnant.

But, asks Buss, why should men bother to get married or commit themselves to a long-term relationship at all? To begin with, men who do not meet the demands of women may not have sex and procreate with the most desirable of females. That is, men, to guarantee their genetic prosperity, have to agree to the terms of sexual mating as laid down by women. Furthermore, there may be an evolutionary requirement for a man to stay with the woman who has borne his children to ensure that they survive both in the physical sense but also to pass on skills and cultural knowledge.

Interestingly, men appear to have an inherent reproductive technique to guard against another man successfully fertilising their partners. Women may be much more indiscriminate about who they have sexual congress with, and how many times they indulge in intercourse in order to get pregnant, than is suggested by Buss' account of evolutionary processes. Robin Baker (1996) has argued that some spermatozoa have the specific function of attacking the sperm of other men inside the woman's reproductive tract. The occurrence of what he describes as 'the sperm wars' suggests that the biology of men has developed in response to female infidelity.

Far from adapting a biological-deterministic stance, Buss as an evolutionist is unusual in that he argues for change in human sexual behaviour. He concludes:

> We are the first species in the known history of three and a half billion years of life on earth with the capacity to control our own destiny. The prospect of designing our destiny remains excellent to the degree that we comprehend our evolutionary past. Only by examining the complex repertoire of human sexual struggles can we know where we came from. Only by understanding why these human strategies have evolved can we control where we are going.
>
> (Buss 1994: 222)

Buss's conviction that humans have the capability to consciously revise their conduct leads him to suggest that contemporary barriers to sexual contentment can be resolved. For example, our evolutionary legacy should not leave us unable to tackle rape, sexism, divorce, the 'sex war' between men and women, sexual disease and human unhappiness in general. Social scientists have, of course, pointed out that both human cognition and the social environment have already altered the effect of biological imperatives.

Superimposed onto these biological impulses is the personal and interpersonal realm which in most cases mediates raw sexuality. Personal choice over sexual partners and forms (if any) of sexual expression, issues of self-awareness and confidence, the availability of willing partners with whom to consort, and the comprehension of what to do when the opportunity to have sex arises, influence our biological urges. Moreover, the high divorce rate, increasing numbers of single-parent families, growing appreciation of emotional and physical abuse in families, occurrence of infidelity, and the pro-active development of a 'singles' way of life (especially amongst young women), indicates that human mating is not only convoluted, defective and painful for many, but also evolutionarily maladaptive.

Overlaying both the biological and personal–interpersonal realms is the cultural domain. The biochemical effect on human sexuality is not in dispute. However, the cultural norms of a society, whilst reflexively affected by the sexual innovation of individuals, fashion how biology becomes behaviour and the boundaries of human inventiveness. It has become a truism that since the 1960s in the West there has been a cultural revolution with respect to sexuality. What is accepted as within a 'normal' range of sexual behaviour in the twenty-first century differs greatly from what was publicly determined as condonable in the nineteenth century and early part of the twentieth century. Up until that time, Judaeo-Christian religion, and then Victorian morality codes, had constructed what we might now refer to as a prudish model of sexuality. During Victorian times, sex also became medicalised with certain sexual behaviours viewed by doctors as forms of madness. For example, excessive self-pleasuring was constructed as 'mastur-batory insanity', and homosexuality was a specific sexual deviancy within a large itinerary of deviancies and perversions requiring psychiatric intervention.

This does not mean that people a century ago were not indulging in a wide range of sexual practices, or that there are now no forms of sexuality left that cannot be carried out and spoken about without public admonition. Although the clitoris and 'G' spot have become notorious since the 1960s, this should not be taken as meaning that no one knew what or where they were in the 1950s. Since the Roman and Greek civilisations sex in all its configurations has been indulged in by sections of all cultures.

Masturbation, oral sex, and, although to a lesser degree, anal sex (involving either homosexuals or heterosexuals), are today not viewed as uncommon or abhorrent. It is worth noting however, that there remains in the twenty-first century much ambiguity and double standards about sexuality. In the USA oral sex is illegal in the states of Maryland, Louisiana and in Washington DC. In these areas fellatio and cunnilingus are held to be 'unnatural carnal copulation'. In Minnesota and Georgia it is illegal for unmarried couples to fornicate. If a married woman has sex with a single man in Idaho she is committing a felony. In most states bestial relations with even a fish are outlawed, except in Wyoming which has no specific statute concerning the issue (Joannides and Gross 1999).

However, there has been also a 'commodification' of sex. That is, from the post-modernist perspective the meaning of sex has been transformed. It has shifted from a mixture of procreation and pleasure, to a concentration on pleasure. The pleasure connotations of sex have then been commandeered by the marketing industry, which has created a vast number of 'sex consumers'.

> An ever expanding range of commodities is sold by invoking sexual imagery, while sexual desirability is increasingly pre- sented as a leisure commodity to be acquired and utilized, whether in relation to self or others. We live, in short, in a sexualised world.

> (Hawkes 1996: 1)

Sexual imagery is used openly to advertise any and every commer- cial product. Symbols of sexuality adorn the covers of books and videos, and feature in the promotion of cinema. Advertisements for cars, toothpaste and ice-cream use sexuality blatantly. Sex scenes are included in films and television programmes to increase the viewing audience. Sex (for example, in the form of pornography) is available extensively on the Internet. There is also a combination of 'sex' and 'health' imagery used to sell popular magazines. Healthiness is sold as sexiness and vice versa both in the advertising of these products and in much of the content.

Sex has always been for sale to men through prostitution, but there is a growth in 'male escort' services for women. Sex toys sold on the basis of aiding sexual pleasure are obtainable widely, and in Britain have become available on the high street through specialist retail outlets. It is not hyperbole to claim that there is an obsession with sex in contemporary society. There has been a move from sex as 'production' (in the sense of making babies) to sex as 'consump- tion' (i.e. it is sold as a product).

The reconstructing and commercialisation of sexuality, however, have brought dramatic shifts in, and what could be considered to be major benefits to, the sexual culture of Western countries. Female sexuality has become recognised and, from an interactionist standpoint, given 'meaning' by the relevant social players – women. From a feminist viewpoint, there has been a notable move towards women's sexual emancipation since the 1960s. In part this has been the payoff from advances in contraception, but it is also because the discourse of sexuality has been made public.

Nancy Friday is an arch proponent of the need to acknowledge and understand women's sexual desires, and has caused much controversy over her publication of fantasies as told to her by respondents who replied to a request for details about what women day-dream about. The late Jill Tweedie, one of the foremost British feminists of the twentieth century, novelist and journalist, has a foreword to Friday's (1976) sexually explicit book *My Secret Garden*. In this foreword Tweedie remarks that Friday's book, apart from being very erotic, is both fascinating and liberating. For Tweedie women's sexual imagination had been, up until this book was written, 'laid underground', and the book is a dramatic provocation to male assumptions that women (unless they are nymphomaniacs or prostitutes) 'lie back and think of England' when engaged in sexual activity.

In a later book, *Women on Top*, Friday lays the blame squarely on male sexism and patriarchy for the historical stifling of women's sexuality:

> It is a patriarchal society that needed, for its establishment and survival, to believe in male sexual supremacy, or more exactly, women's asexuality. How could man wage his wars, put his shoulder to the industrial wheel if half his brain feared that he was being cuckolded, that the little woman was at home – or worse, not at home – satisfying her insatiable lust?
>
> (Friday 1991: 9)

Moreover, achieving sexual contentment has become a goal similar to the attainment of love, good employment and wealth. Sexual knowledge is no longer confined to a few pages in an anatomy and physiology textbook, or to the 'top shelf' pornographic magazines. Nor does it rely on the very unreliable method of 'word-of-mouth' initiated in the school playground. Hundreds if not thousands of sex manuals have been produced describing and illustrating the best techniques for gaining more from sex. Some of these manuals are comprehensive in their content with regard to sexuality, and go far beyond simply instructing the reader on how to achieve, or give, an orgasm. For example, in *The Guide to Getting It On*, written by Paul Joannides and illustrated by Daerick Gross (1999), the following subjects are covered: kissing; nakedness; massage; male and female genitals; self-eroticism and mutual masturbation; sexual inter-course; anal eroticism; vibrators and dildos; talking about sex to a partner; sexual fantasies and dreams; having sex if you are disabled; sex during and after pregnancy; birth control and sexual disease; circumcision; impotency; cross-cultural views on sex; sex on the side of the road.

The sex manual industry is no doubt part of the commodification of sexuality and a cultural edifice of the Western world. However, other cultures have produced explicit guides to sex (for example, the *Kama Sutra*) in the past. Moreover, the display of sexuality and intricate detailing of sexual practices is a sign of the tremendous movement in cultural norms since the Victorian period.

However, not only are there contradictions within Western culture concerning sexuality, but the relative conservativeness of a Judaeo-Christian and medicalised value system compared with, for example, Buddhist beliefs, is stark:

> Buddhists and members of other Eastern cultures make sexuality a part of their religion. They view sex as an important blending of energies that helps with one's spiritual transformation. Many of their most sacred shrines and altars show pictures of people having sex, and they sometimes speak of finding God through getting it on. Here in the West, sex is also an important part of religion. Everything that's bad is at one time or another blamed on sex. You get the feeling that sex was invented by the devil himself.
>
> (Joannides and Gross 1999: 386)

Darwin couldn't have predicted the effect of contraception on the yield of children by the physically and socially privileged. Those that are, in Darwin's words, 'best fitted for their places in nature' (the healthy middle classes) now have far fewer progeny than those who are evolutionarily and socially less desirable. Moreover, Darwin could not have had an inkling that by the twentieth century society would produce 'designer sex' through the development of new reproductive technologies and sexual performance-enhancing drugs. 'In vitro fertilisation' (an ovum or sperm is donated to a woman), surrogate motherhood (one woman carries another's baby), the cloning of human tissue, and Viagra, are changing the ways in which humans procreate. Sex could in the future become entirely recreational.

Equally, the neo-Darwinians have failed to incorporate the effect of the sexual revolution on the mating game. Human engagement with sexual pleasure is a cognitive and cultural imposition on evolutionary theories. If the destruction of patriarchy, and erotic enlightenment, can come about by raising political and sexual consciousness, then biology is an 'also ran' in the race that is human development.

Despite the fascination about homosexuality in the press, as a consequence of some politician or film star being 'outed' as gay, the discovery of a 'gay gene', or the consequence of the gay civil rights groups drawing attention to their cause, and the upsurge of gay and lesbian scholarship, sex for most people involves either only themselves (i.e. through masturbation and other auto-erotic habits) or members of the opposite sex. That is, heterosexuality is the dominant form of sexual expression. However, Judith Lorber (1994) has suggested that far from there only being heterosexuals and homosexuals, there exists a multitude of sexual tastes. Specifically, these are: heterosexual men; heterosexual women; gay men; lesbian women; bisexual men; bisexual women; transvestite men (men who dress as women); transvestite women (women who dress as men); transsexual men (men whose genitalia has been altered to that of a female); transsexual women (women whose genitalia has been altered to that of a male).

Moreover, some of those belonging to one category will veer into another category at some stage in their lives. It is also the case that an unknown number of people opt for celibacy, or cannot find any sexual outlet to their liking. More disturbingly, a few choose to focus on animals to gain sexual satisfaction (bestiality). What is repugnant morally throughout the modern Western world is paedophilia, the sexual consorting of adults with children. However offensive to our codes of right and wrong sexual relations between the legally young and adults may be, historically and cross-culturally there are examples of such practices being normalised (Foucault 1985; Giddens 1997).

Gender

People in human societies are separated into one of two sexes, i.e. either 'male' or female'. Biology dictates the sex of an individual. The external genitals and internal organs of reproduction we have, our facial characteristics and physique, are decreed by biology. However, the sex chromosomes we inherit (XX for a woman and XY for a man) provide only a foundation for sexual identity. Society can be remarkably effective in altering the biological impetus for conduct. 'Gender' is the term used by social scientists to distinguish between an individual's biological make-up and her or his socially constructed sex-role behaviour.

Individuals may choose to live their lives in a gender role that is in direct contradiction to their biological identity. A man may dress and behave as a woman, and a woman as a man, because he or she 'feels' more comfortable in this (opposite) gender role. An operation to change the genitalia to that of the preferred sex may be undertaken. Whilst the sex chromosomes remain the same, this can help the person who is reconstructing her or his gender to play out the adopted character (including experiencing sexuality) more effectively.

The extent to which biology and society each influence the ways in which we act as men and women is debatable. This issue raises questions about how much of what we are as humans is dictated by 'nature' or by the learning processes we are exposed to during our lifetime which 'nurture' our behaviour. Do particular chromosomes and biochemicals enforce a 'masculine' performance for men which involves aggression, an ability to hunt (in pre-industrial times), till the soil (in agrarian economies), or earn a living from wage-labouring or running a business (in capitalist systems)? Do the genetic and hormonal arrangements of women convey the 'feminine' qualities of passivity, cooking, house-cleaning and child-rearing? Does nature determine the reality of being a man means that you die younger than a woman?

One biological fact that does denote specific gender-role behaviours is that women become pregnant, have babies and in the main take on the greater share of caring for their offspring as well as the home. Although fertilised ova can be placed in men's abdominal cavities so that an (artificial) male-pregnancy can be created, and house-husbandry has become a variation on traditional family life, these events are still novelties. Women are usually constrained in what they can achieve in the workplace and in their social lives because of their reproductive capacity.

However, this is not necessarily the outcome of biology, but of the social environment in which reproduction takes place. It is society that expects women to concentrate on being a 'mother' and a 'wife' (and to fulfil the obligation of working part-time). In situations where child-care facilities allow women to engage fully with their careers and out-of-work pursuits, biology takes second place to social determinants.

Moreover, with reference to hormones, violence has become linked to higher levels of testosterone in men compared with women, and excessive amounts found in some men. This is seen as primary evidence for the case of nature affecting (male) behaviour. However, as Giddens (1997) suggests, the conclusions that can be reached from studies into male aggression amongst monkeys are ambiguous:

> Research has indicated, for instance, that if male monkeys are castrated at birth, they become less aggressive; conversely, female monkeys given testosterone will become more aggressive than normal females. However, it has also been found that providing monkeys with opportunities to dominate others actually increases the testosterone level. Aggressive behaviour may thus affect the production of the hormone, rather than the hormone causing increased aggression.
>
> (Giddens 1997: 92)

It would be rare to find the opportunity to replicate this research in humans. Finding men who are willing to undergo such a study is doubtful (and highly unethical), and finding enough to conduct a randomised control trial is even more improbable. Therefore, we have to be cautious about what conclusions can be drawn from animal studies when considering human behaviour.

Helman (1994) suggests that an individual's gender can be assessed on the basis of four elements. First, there is the underlying 'genotypical' formation (i.e. the sex chromosomes). Second, there are the 'phenotypical' secondary-sex characteristics (i.e. appearance and body shape). Third, there is the psychological aspect (i.e. an individual's self-perception and understanding of her or his sexual identity). Fourth, there are cultural perceptions (i.e. norms of society that place pressure on an individual to dress, talk and think in ways that are regarded as appropriate to a sex role).

There is interplay between these elements, with one or more dominating the others in any particular individual. For example, the influence of culture in advanced industrial societies is probably heightened compared to societies made up of hunters and gatherers. In the latter type of society, genotype and phenotype sexual distinctions are more likely to be prominent in guiding behaviour and forming social expectations. Furthermore, individualism is more in accord with capitalist ideology, so that if a man wishes to act as a woman this is perhaps not only tolerated but his needs will be commodified and a market in 'cross-dressing' will follow.

Moreover, habits alter within a gender and are interchangeable between genders, as a consequence in shifts of cultural expectations. For example, certain civilisations have tolerated behaviours in both men and women that in other epochs are not viewed as befitting to the gender in question. In Elizabethan times, it was thought masculine for men to wear cod-pieces, thereby accentuating the size of their sexual organs. Apart from perhaps a small number of rock music artists, this practice is defunct and would now attract ridicule. Women a few decades ago would not have worn trousers, whereas these days they are a regular feature of feminine dress. The performance of strip-tease has historically been considered a female craft for the delectation of men. Strip-tease by men now attracts huge female audiences.

Changes in cultural patterns can have a dramatic effect on sexual performance generally, and on the individual's psychological comprehension of her or his own sexuality. In certain middle-eastern countries, African and pre-industrial societies male homosexuality is taken as the norm, and in many Western countries a much more broad-minded view has developed to both male and female homosexuality. Moreover, a heterosexual woman or man may find that, being placed in, for example, a single-sex environment for a long period of time (such as a prison) may sway her or his sexual leanings towards homosexuality.

In Greco-Roman culture, heterosexuality was not given a higher status than homosexuality (Foucault 1985). Men indulged in sexual acts with women, slaves and boys. Pleasures of the flesh (eating, drinking and fornicating) were thought to be vital human dispositions. Indulging in these hedonistic activities was believed necessary to appease the pagan gods. However, it was the loss of control during sexual encounters that men in classical antiquity feared, and hence they had to be seen to be dominant in their sexual relations. Activity was, for ancient Greek and Roman men, 'natural' and indicated virility (Hawkes 1996). What they despised was such inert acts as performing fellatio and cunnilingus and being penetrated rather than being the penetrator. It was not homosexuality that was decreed abnormal but passivity.

However, in other societies homosexuality has been viewed as morally repugnant, and may be legally forbidden. In some states in the USA homosexuality is a crime for which the perpetrator can technically be given a prison sentence. This was also the case until the 1990s in the Australian state of Tasmania. The legal infringement of 'buggery' in England and Wales until 1861, whether involving other men, women or animals, carried the death penalty (Hawkes 1996).

Indeed, the willing participation by adults in certain sexual acts is no protection from the law. In 1992 a group of sado-masochistic homosexual men, who had in private whipped, cut and branded each other over a ten-year period (none of whom suffered any permanent injury) were found guilty in an English court of 'Offences Against the Person'. They were also to lose an appeal to the House of Lords on the basis that it was not in the public interest for people to cause bodily harm to each other for no good reason (Geary 1998).

Helman (1994) also records how there are genotype discrepancies that undermine the simple division of humans into men and women. Specifically, sex chromosome abnormalities may result in hermaphroditism whereby both male and female constituents are present, Turner's syndrome in which there is only one X chromosome, or Klinefelter's syndrome whose sufferers have the combination of XXY. These conditions are unusual. More exceptional, but very instructive in demonstrating that splitting humans into two gender categories is problematic, is the situation where there is a discrepancy between an individual's genotypology and phenotypology. That is, a few people are born with chromosomes belonging to one sex, but the genitalia that pertains to the other.

The socialisation process allows the culture of a society to inculcate an individual's way of behaving in her or his gender role. That is, the norms, values, mores, beliefs and practices of that society related to masculinity or femininity are passed on to the individual through his or her family and close friends. Research into how parents react to their babies demonstrates that males and females are treated very differently (Giddens 1997). Babies are given divergent clothes, toys and books dependent on their biological sex; are spoken to in alternative ways; and handled either roughly or gently on the basis of whether they are a boy or a girl.

Significant others, apart from members of her or his primary socialisation group, also pass on messages about how to carry out appropriate gender conduct. Secondary socialisation takes place with contact being made more outside of the family. Teachers and fellow pupils, and those with whom the individual shares her or his social life, will reaffirm acceptable patterns of role behaviour for females and males. The media, the Internet, films and video games, however, have become forcible socialisation instruments. Many of the signals about gender received from these sources may contradict previous messages. Media and electronic communications may open the individual up to alternative ways of enacting gender roles.

Referring specifically to sexual intercourse, but by implication making a general point about sexuality, Kate Millett in her book *Sexual Politics* makes the following observation:

> Coitus can scarcely be said to take place in a sexual vacuum; although of itself it appears as a biological and physical activity, it is set so deeply within the larger context of human affairs that it serves as a charged microcosm of the variety of attitudes and values to which culture subscribes.
>
> (Millett 1977: 23)

Millett's (feminist) stance is that power-relationships between men and women are reified in the sexual act. Men copulate with women with the same domineering intention they enact in other spheres of male–female contact. But Robert Connell (1996) argues that there is no one male role that each man adopts, but many 'masculinities'. Hence, the feminist stereotyping of men as exploiters of women and contributors to a patriarchal social structure belies the divergent patterns of behaviour that can be found amongst men. Some men subjugate women, but some women abuse men. Many men do not engage at all in this power struggle with women. Moreover, men from different social categories have very contrary role behaviours, and may have more in common with the norms displayed by women in the same group than with their gender counterparts from other sections of society.

In an examination of gender representations from ancient to modern, Thomas Lacquer has argued that during the medieval epoch the assumption was that there was only one gender – the male. The existence of male genitalia was viewed as indicating a complete human. Women, therefore, were regarded as incomplete men rather than belonging to an opposite or different gender group. This consideration of women being 'sub-human' or 'inferior' men, of course, has its antecedent in Judaeo-Christian beliefs about Eve being made from the (spare) rib of Adam. Moreover, Victorian attitudes towards female genitalia (i.e. perceiving them as indicating emotional weakness) contributed to explications of women's psychological maladies that persisted into twentieth-century psychiatric theory. For example, early psychiatric interpretations of mental illnesses with signs of physical impairment laid the blame on the existence of the uterus. 'Hysteria', is derived from the Greek word *hystero*, meaning womb.

The seminal research of Alfred Kinsey, which began in the 1930s and continued into the 1950s, was to produce a taxonomy of human sexual habits that demolished the Victorian and medical separation of behaviour into 'normal' and 'abnormal'. He did not accept, for example, that people were either 'heterosexual' or 'homosexual' (Kinsey *et al.* 1948; 1953). He argued that individuals may have heterosexual or homosexual experiences which were indicative of what they enjoyed, but this did not reflect a specific type of constitution. Consequently, Kinsey was in favour of viewing sexuality on a continuum, which may have heterosexuality at one end and homosexuality at the other. However, this continuum has branches that lead to forms of sexual expression that cannot be categorised as either heterosexual or homosexual. Moreover, the results from his studies contested the Judaeo-Christian moral convention that people should not (or did not) indulge in sexual outlets unless married, and then only with their married partner.

His sampling of white American men and women was to cause outrage. What Kinsey discovered in his surveys was that not only were the unmarried people of white America pursing diverse and regular methods of sexual release (from masturbation to bestiality), but well over a third of the male population at some time in their lives admitted to having had a significant homosexual experience. At least 17 per cent of women had also been brought to orgasm by other women. Nearly all men reported that they masturbated, as did a majority of women. Clearly, masturbation could not any longer be construed as exceptional, unnatural or unhealthy.

Risks

As Helman (1994) records, the norms of a society influence patterns of sexual behaviour, which in turn affect rates of venereal disease. Gonorrhoea, syphilis, genital herpes and AIDS are more common in societies that accept sexual promiscuity, sex outside marriage, prostitution (for men) and homosexuality. There is in these societies literally more opportunity to get and pass on the responsible germs, and for epidemics to be transmitted quickly and to a large number of people. The price for sexual freedom is sexual disease, unless a vulnerable society or community within a particular social system, is educated in, and practices, 'safe sex'. Those societies that do not control sexuality through moral codes or legislation, and whose citizens do not practise safe sex or have access to antibiotics and anti-viral drugs, are especially susceptible to unbridled disease.

Gender behaviour also leads to ill-health (Helman 1994). For men, adherence to the conventional masculine role (which involves aggression, stoicism and competitiveness) is linked to being a victim of violent crime, the avoidance of medical help until a disease or disability is well established, alcoholism, accidents in sports and at work, work-related stress and coronary heart disease. For women, their traditional role of domesticity and the expectation to remain youthful and physically admirable, can lead to depression and eating disorders and surgical intervention to alter body shape (with the inherent dangers of botched operations and death during anaesthesia).

The reoccurrence of sex diseases that had been previously controlled, and/or the establishment of new sex diseases may rebound on sexual liberation. We have become obsessed with risk due to the apparent uncertainties of modern life (Beck 1992). Calculations of probability are made about dying from cancer, crashing in an aeroplane as a result of computer failure, contracting a sexually transmitted disease, winning the lottery and living longer by drinking red wine (Giddens 1999). Although the incidence of most of the main sex diseases of old have grown steadily, it is the materialisation of novel conditions such as genital herpes and especially AIDS, and its precursory stage of infection by the human immunodeficiency virus (HIV), that has heightened levels of anxiety in the mating game. Such anxieties could result in a return to the sexual mores that have been associated with the Victorian era.

However, it is debatable how much the risk of contracting such a serious if not fatal disease has altered patterns of sexual behaviour. A joint *Guardian*/ICM poll on sexual morality was conducted in Britain during December of 1999, and the results compared with polls undertaken in 1955 and 1969 (Travis 1999). The 1999 poll used a random sample of over 1,000 people over eighteen years old, and was carried out by telephone. The conclusion reached by the pollsters was that, whilst overall people were far more liberal in their views compared to those reported in the earlier studies (especially towards the acceptability of sex before marriage and of cohabitation), there was a conspicuous difference between adults aged twenty-four and under, and those in the twenty-five years to sixty-four years group. Younger people were much less likely to approve of sex before commitment to a long-term relationship, and were less approving of the use of the contraceptive pill – the device that had been so advantageous to their parents' generation in allowing sexual pleasure without the pressure of involuntary reproduction. But, in a number of African countries, the massive rise in the number of people with HIV infection, and those dying of AIDS, and the apparent increase in people affected in China, suggest that any actual alteration in sexual habits (for example, less partners; the use of condoms during intercourse; a lesser reliance on penetrative sex whether this is vaginal, anal or oral) is sporadic.

The discovery of genital herpes in the 1970s commanded a media panic about risk from this incurable but not fatal infection. It was dubbed in the press 'the new sexual leprosy', and tens of millions in the USA alone were thought to carry the infection. By 1981, however, the first cases of AIDS were found in the USA, a disease that was both debilitating and lethal. There was justification for the media attention, and medical and public concern that this 'new plague' attracted. AIDS spread quickly, and by the 1990s could deservedly be described as a world-wide epidemic that was out of control.

However, AIDS, due to its mode of transmission, has been selective in which sections of the population and which communities it has targeted. It has hit mainly those who are already socially stigmatised and marginalised – drug users, homosexuals, poor communities. Virginia van der Vliet argues also that in each society in which AIDS was portrayed as a threat to the 'normal' population (i.e. heterosexual middle classes), the disease was constructed in culturally relevant ways. Constructions usually involved blaming the victims, or scapegoating groups seen to threaten social stability or the interests of other sections of society:

in each place the disease was given a 'social construction' – it assimilated the meanings, the anxieties and the prejudices of that time and place. In the United States fears of changing sexual mores allowed homophobia to re-emerge as a fear of AIDS. In France and elsewhere in Europe, threats of job losses to waves of new immigrants revived old xenophobic attitudes, this time in the guise of fears about foreigners bringing AIDS into the country. In South Africa, fears about a new social order reactivated racism masquerading as concerns about AIDS in desegregated swimming pools and lavatories.

(Vliet 1996: 3)

As Vliet comments, AIDS became known globally as 'divine retribution' for moral decay. It was a plague sent by God as nemesis for the post-1960s' culture of sexual debauchery (exemplified by the growing incidents of pre-marital sex, extra-marital sex, under-age sex, one-parent families and homosexual acts).

However, whilst there has been an undoubted amplification of fear surrounding the threat of AIDS to the general (heterosexual) population, do the facts not bear out a need for the mobilisation of conservative forces if only in order to change sexual behaviour? Does the drama that occurred in the first world, and is now reoccurring in the second and third worlds, not serve the purpose of making governments and international organisations such as WHO and the United Nations rally their resources and focus on geographical and population hot-spots where AIDS appears to be unregulated? Moreover, if the reaction to AIDS is about the powerful denigrating the powerless, as suggested by Vliet, how is the lot of the latter improved by not having the 'gaze' of politicians, journalists, scientists, health promoters and medical practitioners focused on this issue?

In the late 1990s, the United Nations (UN) and WHO produced a joint report on the epidemic of AIDS (UN/WHO 1998). The report stated that throughout the world 30.6 million people had HIV/AIDS at the end of 1997, of whom 1.1 million were children under fifteen years of age. During 1997 there were 5.8 million new cases of HIV/AIDS, and 2.3 million deaths from the disease of whom nearly half a million were children below fifteen years. Since the beginning of the epidemic 11.7 million people had died from AIDS or AIDS-related diseases. The number of children who had by 1997 lost either their mother or both parents because of AIDS was 8.2 million.

HIV/AIDS is one of the ten biggest killer diseases worldwide. The UN and WHO (1998) suggest that unless there is individual and political action (nationally and internationally) aimed at altering sexual behaviour, making available necessary finances for health promotion programmes, and finding a cure, the death toll will rise steadily.

HIV infections are concentrated in the poorest parts of the third world. Nearly 90 per cent of people with HIV live in sub-Saharan Africa, and the developing countries of Asia. The gross national product of these countries is below 10 per cent of that of all the other countries of the world. However, rates of HIV infection are increasing fast in Eastern Europe and China. In these countries it is heterosexual sex, rather than homosexual sex and the use of infected needles (which were the initial causes of spread in the West), that is responsible for the increase in infection.

However, the UN/WHO report suggests that in African countries, where action has been taken to prevent the diffusion of HIV, rates appear to have stabilised or even reduced. For example, the Ugandan government involved traditional healers, community leaders and teachers in a programme aimed at educating young people about unprotected sex, and the dangers of having many sexual partners or of having sex at an early age. Asian countries such as Thailand have also seen a drop in recorded HIV infection. The Thai government focused on educating sex workers (who were not just passing on the disease to fellow citizens but also to the substantial number of 'sex tourists' from other parts of the world) in cities such as Bangkok.

HIV rates seem to be on the way down in Europe and the USA. This is largely seen as a consequence of gay communities taking the initiative by advocating alternative sexual practices from unprotected anal sex. Moreover, heterosexual young men have been encouraged by government-sponsored advertising campaigns to use condoms to protect themselves. There are exceptions, however. For example, there was an increase of over 30 per cent in new cases of AIDS among black Americans, and nearly 20 per cent among Hispanics.

So, there remain structural discrepancies between sections of society, and areas of the world. These structural issues, concerning poverty, education and access to medical treatment, need to be addressed. The danger is not that nothing can be done about AIDS, but that when an epidemic occurs in places or communities that are not a major concern, either directly or indirectly, for Western governments, people will be left to solve their own problems. Although it is possible that some affected groups will take up the challenge and be effective in stemming the disease (as has happened with the gay communities of the West and governments of countries such as Uganda), others will be left to rot due to their political, cultural and economic irrelevance to the West, and/or the lack of the media spotlight on them.

Summary

Sexuality, gender and sexual disease, are major and complex social issues. Although there are signs that there is some degree of retrenchment over what is considered to be acceptable sexual behaviour, how society regards sex has changed remarkably in a relatively short period of time. Sexual variety, both in terms of practices and identities, is in general tolerated in contemporary society.

Whilst the debate about how much of gender behaviour is determined by 'nature' or 'nurture' persists, male and female sexuality appears to cross the boundaries of role-specific styles. That is, there are many 'sexualities', and these may not be confined to one gender or another.

Sex, however, brings risk. Disease caught through sexual contact is responsible for the deaths of millions of people throughout the world. Nurses could be at the forefront of health movements that aim not only to alter sexual behaviours, but the social conditions that help to create such outrageous loss of life

Further reading

Hawkes, G. (1996) *A Sociology of Sex and Sexuality*, Buckingham: Open University Press.

Chapter 9

Madness

Madness is everywhere. Nurses, doctors and other health-care workers come across madness throughout their careers. This may be in the specialist area of mental health (where the health-care worker may be on 'placement' during training, or is employed permanently) or whilst working in a hospital or in primary care. Accident and emergency departments and general practitioner surgeries abound with madness. The mental health worker, operating in a very stressful area of care delivery, may herself or himself suffer a 'mental health problem' (a modern-day euphemism for madness). It is highly unlikely that she or he has not had a mad loved-one or relative, although in the past this may have been a family secret with the affected person mysteriously concealed from view and perhaps institutionalised beyond the gaze of 'normal' society. But what is madness?

Mad definitions

In Britain a survey of the incidence of psychiatric symptoms, using a sample of 10,000 adults living in private households, found that one in seven adults aged between sixteen years and sixty-four years had a 'neurotic' illness during one specified week (Meltzer *et al.* 1994). The researchers reported that women were much more likely to suffer from neurosis, but that men suffered from alcohol and drug dependency in far greater numbers. Fatigue, disturbed sleep, irritability and worry were found to be the most common symptoms of mental disorder, with anxiety and depression the most prevalent disorders.

Up to 30 per cent of Australians may have a mental disorder, and 3 per cent of the population can be described as being seriously mentally ill (Hazelton 1999). In the USA it has been estimated that each year nearly a third of the population experiences one form or another of madness, with nearly 2 per cent having a serious disorder (Cockerham 1996). Nearly half of USA citizens may have symptoms of a mental disorder at some point in their lives. So many USA citizens receive psychiatric help that the country has been described as the 'therapeutic society'.

Measurements of ill-health used by the World Health Organisation (WHO), which include not just mortality rates but the social cost of premature deaths and morbidity, have indicated that the real burden of psychiatric illness in Western countries accounts for more than that of heart disease and cancer (WHO 1999). Such a calculation encompasses the human and financial cost of madness in terms of individual suffering, the distressing effect on families and communities, and the percentage of gross national product spent on services.

A figure of $67 billion for one year (1992) has been estimated as the direct expenditure for treating mental disorder in the United States (Cockerham 1996). It has been suggested that in Britain the financial burden of mental disorder is greater than that of the defence budget, and represents 4 per cent of the gross domestic product. The calculation of £32 billion (for the year 1996–97) by health economists at the Institute of Psychiatry in London, is based on adding together the figures for: wasted productivity (including that lost through suicide); social security payments, health, local authority and criminal justice services; and informal care (Brindle 1997).

But defining what the condition of madness is, and what its boundaries are, is extremely problematic, and to a large extent depends on who is asking the questions. It also depends upon what notions of normality are being adopted at the time in that particular place, and whether or not there are identifiable behaviours and thoughts that are universally describable as so strange (i.e. abnormal) to warrant the tag of madness.

Mad people everywhere are segregated from 'normal' people, either physically (i.e. they are put in institutions) or socially (i.e. they are excluded from sharing life experiences with the rest of the population). The basis for the segregation is 'strangeness'. The mad are regarded as behaving and/or thinking differently to the rest of the population. This strangeness may be regarded as self-threatening or signalling danger to others. Individuals affected by strangeness might not be taking care of themselves (for example, neglecting personal hygiene, and not eating), or could be suicidal or homicidal. An assessment of strangeness may be made by the sufferer (who asks for help from family, friends or from 'professionals' such as the shaman, priest or psychotherapist). Alternatively, assistance to become normal may be thrust upon those detected as abnormal by the agencies of social control such as the police, social services, psychiatry and psychiatric nursing.

However, lots of 'normal' people have beliefs that are similar to those of the mad, and behave comparably. Suicide and violence is not confined to the mad. Non-mad people can decide to take their own lives, perhaps as a consequence of severe pain from a chronic illness, or a complete lack of hope in the future due to particular social circumstances. Football fans, drunks and young men have a history of aggression that far outstrips that of the mad. Certain people (i.e. soldiers and spies) are given licence to kill by the State. Students are notorious for being unkempt and living frugally. Anyone who has religious beliefs, or who considers astrology a predictive body of knowledge, could be described as having mad thoughts. Why is there selectivity over who is condoned as mad when there is so much strangeness in society?

There are essentially two interpretations that can be made about why certain behaviours and thoughts by particular people are deemed to be either so strange, or are of a particular type of strangeness, that they merit an identity of 'madness'. The first is that propounded by the *mad doctors* (and by association, the 'mad nurses'). The second is in direct competition with the first, and offers social explanations of madness.

Whilst distinguishable from each other, neither the first nor the second interpretation is internally consistent. There are many disagreements between the mad doctors about what is and what causes madness, and what treatments can be effective. Likewise, there is a wide divergence of views from the proponents of socially generated madness. In general, however, mad doctors regard the mad individual as the locus for both aetiology and management, whereas sociologists argue that even if society isn't the origin of madness then the way in which it is organised still needs to be taken into account in order to understand what might precipitate the condition and how it should be treated.

Just to add to the complexity of the subject of madness, however, some mad doctors deliver 'social' therapy through which there is an integration of personal issues with family and work-related factors. Psychiatric nursing, whilst remaining connected strongly to scientific medicine and empirical evidence, does embrace its alternative gurus and faiths. Moreover, a number of those who concentrate on the structure and culture of society in their search for the meaning of madness, accept mental disorder as a fact (in the positivist sense). Others in the social madness camp deny that madness exists at all, but aim to supply remedies to the disabling effects of madness by exorcising stigmatising labels, and chastening those who do the labelling.

Similarly, the programmes of care or containment directed at those displaying strangeness are discrepant. The bizarre conduct of the insane is analogous to the 'mad policies' of successive governments.

Mad doctors

> What was it like to live in a world without psychiatry? In Ireland it was like this: In 1817, a member of the House of Commons from an Irish district said: 'There is nothing so shocking as madness in the cabin of the Irish peasant. ... When a strong man or woman gets the complaint, the only way they have to manage is by making a hole in the floor of the cabin, not high enough for the person to stand up in, with a crib over it to prevent his getting up. The hole is about five feet deep, and they give this wretched being his food there, and there he generally dies'.
>
> (Shorter 1997: 1–2)

In the West, the ascendant explanation of madness has emanated from the profession of medicine. That is, madness is construed explicitly as a 'disorder' or 'illness' akin to physical ailments, and is 'treated' by doctors specialising in the subject. Western medicine portrays a world without psychiatry as one of mistaken beliefs, cruelty and devoid of effective care.

Psychiatry posits that its epistemological tenets can be applied to all peoples, in all cultures, throughout time. Whether madness is described as 'Amok' (Malaysia), 'Pibloktoq' (the Arctic), 'Bena Bena' (New Guinea), 'Imu' (Japan), 'Koro' (China), 'Windigo Psychosis' (native North Americans), or 'schizophrenia' (Britain, USA, Europe, Australasia), it is considered by Western psychiatrists to be the same entity. Witchcraft in medieval Europe was merely unrecognised psychosis. The spiritual commands of Saint Michael,

Saint Catherine and Saint Margaret to the French patriot Jeannne d'Arc in the fifteenth century, the delusional symptoms of the crazed.

But psychiatry as an arm of medicine is a European invention. Much of the historical accounting of psychiatry focuses on developments in Britain. Lucy Johnstone (1989) has reviewed what she describes as the conventional history of British psychiatry. This is the version whereby psychiatrists promote the idea that, although there have been failures and successes in the treatment of the mentally disordered, the general direction is one of greater understanding of causation, much more effective treatments, and a far more humane and liberal philosophy of care. The late eighteenth and early nineteenth century was a time in which supernatural explanations of madness were displaced by the scientific exegeses of a medical profession that now encompassed psychiatry within its training. Treatments at this stage are still rudimentary, but were displacing gradually the medieval stage of 'irrational' celestial management which was often mediated through such religious symbols as holy water:

> With those thought to be possessed, treatment was spiritual in intent even if it took a physical form. Belief in the power of holy water to cleanse the soul meant that lunatics were not infrequently bathed or suddenly ducked in a source thought to be holy. In the case of unexpected immersions in water, the procedure may well have been influenced by the observation that shock seemed to render some lunatics more sensible, at least temporarily. Other uses of holy water included the practice of blinding madmen and madwomen, sprinkling them with water from a holy source, and then leaving them to sleep.
>
> (Andrews *et al.* 1997: 102)

Although since the fifteenth century institutions for the mad had been provided (Bethlem, the oldest psychiatric institution in Europe had offered sanctuary from the 1400s onwards: Andrews *et al.* 1997), the mad were in the main still cared for by their families before the nineteenth century. However, thousands of mentally disordered people were contained, from the seventeenth century onwards, within houses of correction, private madhouses and local parish workhouses.

Following the 1845 Lunacy Act in England, local authorities were forced to provide for the mad through a massive public building programme. Asylums were to house more than 100,000 inmates by 1900. The orthodox version of psychiatric history views the asylums as necessary for the protection of the mad and to offer them a decent habitat and appropriate (for the time) medical treatment for the duration of their illness.

But the people who promoted the building of asylums during the Victorian era were in general not medical practitioners but local philanthropists and magistrates. Undoubtedly, the insane institution was a forbidding and oppressive place to spend years if not all of one's remaining life if committed there, and some inmates faced deplorable 'care' at the hands of their keepers and doctors:

> In 1812, scandal broke when Godfrey Higgins discovered in York Asylum (of which he was governor) thirteen women in a cell twelve feet by seven feet ten inches, and that the deaths of 144 patients had been concealed. The same spring, Edward Wakefield found a side-room in Bethlem hospital where ten female patients were chained by one arm or leg to the wall. In a lower gallery (traditionally the area of an asylum where the 'troublesome' and 'dirty' patients were kept), the pitiable figure of James Norris was found, confined to the trough where he lay. Norris died of consumption a few days after his release.
>
> (Fennell 1996: 14)

But brutality had not been expected by the organisers of the asylums. Moreover, given the appalling privations endured by the poor and most working people at the time (Engels 1892), their beneficence is extraordinary. For an individual to be moved away from the squalid existence experienced by those who, from a Marxist perspective, were the casualties of early industrialisation, into an institution where at least food, clothes and reasonable shelter were offered, may not have been the imposition on human freedom that with hindsight we consider it to be.

Furthermore, for many inmates residence in the asylum was a refuge from far worse treatment at the hands of their relatives. Edward Shorter refers to the 'care' received by the mad from their families and the community both in Germany and England in the eighteenth century. He describes such care as a 'horror story'. Moreover, patients received into the asylums were found regularly to be in a terrible state following years of ill-treatment at the hands of their relatives or, in the case of England, the administrators of the institutions for other sorts of social 'deviants' (i.e. the poor). One youth from Wurzurg had been kept in a pig pen by his father, and ate from a bowl by lapping up the food as would an animal. Many of those admitted into the asylums would show signs of having been routinely beaten:

> One [German] man had been chained by his wife to the wall of their house for five years, losing the use of his legs. ... In England, such patients, if not chained at home, might be fastened to a stake in a workhouse or poorhouse.
>
> (Shorter 1997: 3)

The New World was no better. In the USA the pattern was the same, with reports of mentally deranged people being kept by their families in cages, or in stables. Almshouses in Massachusetts contained locked rooms with inadequate ventilation where the mad would be put, sleeping on fouled straw. In Australia, the Fremantle 'round' prison housed the mad in tiny ill-lit stone cells.

Asylums offered the medical specialist the opportunity to deliver and experiment with new treatments. Psychiatric treatments in the nineteenth century involved stimulants, sedatives, emetics, purgatives, bloodletting, cold and hot baths (without the religious overtones), mechanical restraints and electric shocks. However, 'moral treatment', supported by lay benefactors and religious groups such as the Quakers, was to compete with organic medicine. Institutions, for example, the Retreat in York, were built and set up in opposition to those run by medical practitioners (such as the York Asylum). Moral management held that the mad could be brought back to reason if handled more humanely:

> This movement aimed in effect to revive the dormant humanity of the mad, by treating them as endowed with a residuum at least of normal emotions, still capable of excitation and training. ... They needed to be treated essentially like children, who required a stiff dose of rigorous discipline, rectification and retraining in thinking and training.
>
> (Porter 1987: 19)

Employing a technique which has served the profession of medicine extremely well, rather than deriding this popular approach, doctors encompassed moral therapy within their assortment of procedures.

The effect of 'medicalising' moral treatment was to leave psychiatrists 'in charge of the whole enterprise' (Johnstone 1989: 177). From the point of view of the psychiatrists, this move gave their patients the benefit of both scientific treatment and compassionate care.

The Victorian asylums, and those that came after in the twentieth century, were an enormous financial investment for governments of the day, one which could not be replicated today. They were built on the back of high ideals. The mad could partake of fresh air in rural surroundings, in the extensive grounds and gardens that most of the asylums had procured (Gittins 1998). Food and water was comparatively fresh, pure and nutritious. Recreation and rest were encouraged, as was (with the introduction of 'moral therapy') industrious activity when the inmate was perceived to be in need of such to aid her or his recovery.

By the time the 1890 Lunacy Act was instituted, the profession of medicine had monopolised the market with regard to the care of the mad, and this resulted in the redefining of the category of 'madness' to one of 'mental illness'. After 1845, the keeper changed into the 'attendant'. The attendants were responsible for the general upkeep of the new institutions for the insane, but were to become 'the medical superintendent's servants, with primary responsibility to carry out his orders' (Nolan 1993: 6). Women who became attendants were in the main referred to as 'nurses'. At the end of the nineteenth century men were also accorded this title.

A new age of community care arrived in the early part of the twentieth century in Europe and the USA with the mental hygiene movement (Goodwin 1997). Outpatient clinics were established, and further medical treatments developed (for example, insulin therapy and electro-convulsant-therapy). A major achievement for psychiatry in the USA and Europe was the discovery of drugs in the 1950s that could dampen down psychotic symptoms. This, according to the orthodox approach, was nothing short of a revolution in psychiatric care. It allowed previously deranged patients to at least spend large amounts of time 'on leave' or even to be discharged altogether.

Psychiatry, because it had pursued and found through scientific methods, biological causes for some types of madness (specifically, the syphilis generating 'general paralysis of the insane' and senile dementia), and had used with some degree of success chemical therapies, was now firmly clasped within the medical fold. Asylums had become mental 'hospitals', general practitioners offered psycho-pharmaceutical remedies or called in their psychiatric colleagues, and each district general hospital had a department of psychological medicine. The mad and their relatives were assured of a similar quality of treatment given by similarly qualified medical practitioners as was provided to those who suffered from physical ailments.

However, community services were never able to compensate for the loss of many of the large institutions. As a consequence, care in the community has been abandoned as the only policy of choice, and standards in the remaining in-patient services have come under intense criticism. Some of this criticism has been aimed specifically at nurses.

For example, Higgins *et al.* (1999) interviewed over one hundred staff and fifty-two patients, and observed ward activity in eleven sites of acute services. These researchers concluded that the education psychiatric nurses receive does not equip them adequately for working in acute settings. Higgins *et al.* also recorded that the increase in time that senior ward staff spent on paperwork and office duties was 'astonishing'. The most senior of these nurses in 1985 spent a third of their time on this type of work. By 1996, nearly three-quarters of their time was occupied with administrative tasks. These nurses were in direct contact with patients in 1996 for less than 6 per cent of their working day, compared with nearly 30 per cent in 1986. As a consequence:

> many [patients] had only a passing relationship with nurses who were typically in the office writing, telephoning or dealing with unexpected incidents in the ward. This resulted in the boredom reported by many patients who, when in hospital, felt that they were often left to their own devices.
>
> (Higgins *et al.* 1999: 154)

Under the New Labour government's epithet of the 'Third Way', the Department of Health launched its objective to renovate all mental health provision in the late 1990s, reformulating mental health law and establishing guidelines on 'national standards'. Although these changes are presented as a way of avoiding the pitfalls of policies based solely on either the asylum or the community, there is in effect a 'post-liberal' re-emphasis on institutional care and public safety (Morrall 2000). That is, the 'Third Way' gives much more weight to acute in-patient hospital services, secure accommodation and the need to protect both the public and the mentally disordered by removing 'dangerous' patients from the community, rather than being a pledge to re-invest in the policy of care in the community.

Emulating their colleagues in physical medicine, the mad doctors are attracted to diagnostic categories. Psychiatrist Jennifer Hughes extols the virtues of medical categories in her book *An Outline of Modern Psychiatry*:

> A sound classification system is just as desirable in psychiatry as in other branches of medicine. Assigning each case to a recognisable diagnostic category (while continuing to respect the importance of features unique to the patient concerned) has many advantages in clinical work.
>
> (Hughes 1991: 3)

By the start of the third millennium, psychiatry's nosology contained thousands of psychiatric diseases, and a vast array of treatments. Psychiatric medicine has embraced the 'talking therapies' (for example, psychoanalysis, cognitive-behavioural therapy and humanistic counselling). With the arrival of a new wave of anti-depressants and anti-psychotic drugs, and the impending 'cure all' consequences of quantum mechanics and genetic mapping, the mad doctor is better equipped than ever before to eclipse 'discrepant' explanations of strangeness.

The medical profession collaborates with national government health departments and international health organisations in the formulation and distribution of facts and figures about, and classifications of, psychological distress. There are two main classification systems. The first, the International Classification of Diseases, is compiled by WHO. The second is the Diagnostic and Statistical Manual of Mental Disorders of the American Psychiatric Association. Included in both is an extensive list of psychological maladies: organic mental disorders (for example, senile dementia); psychotic disorders (principally schizophrenia); mood disorders (for example, depression and mania); neurotic disorders (for example, anxiety); somatoform disorders (i.e. where physical symptoms, such as paralysis or blindness, are the result of psychological stress); disorders of the personality; disorders involving substance abuse (for example, alcoholism and heroin addiction); eating disorders (for example, anorexia nervosa and bulimia).

However, the fact that there are two systems of classification, and that both regularly revise their contents, suggest that psychiatric diagnosis is not constant and universal. What is deemed to be incorporated in the array of mad behaviours in one year may not be embraced in ensuing eras. Conversely, what is considered to be a normal behaviour or thought today may be reinterpreted as madness tomorrow.

Mad society

The history of madness as presented by the medical profession is one of straightforward scientific development. However, not only do the definitional ambiguities suggest that such an approach is unconvincing, but the availability of a wide range of viewpoints indicates that madness is a contested topic (Coppock and Hopton 2000; Pilgrim and Rogers 1999). In particular, the role of society in the manufacture of madness must be appreciated.

The effect of the social structure on health in general is incontrovertible. For example, the position an individual is situated within the social hierarchy based on class or wealth correlates with chronic disease and mortality. The further down the hierarchy a person is, the more disease-ridden she or he will be, and the earlier death will ensue. Poorer people suffer from psychiatric problems far more than those who are successful (in terms of both financial and cultural capital) in society (Gomm 1996). For example, there is a strong connection between (lower) social class, and alcohol and drug addiction, schizophrenia, depression, Alzheimer's disease and personality disorder. A number of mental disorders occur more frequently amongst those further up the social scale, for example, eating disorders, manic-depression and the anxiety states (Cockerham 1996).

A structuralist position is taken by Andrew Scull (1979; 1984). He refers to the specific role of psychiatry (a branch of the profession of medicine) as an agency of social control which serves the capitalist state by keeping 'the mad' (one section of the proletariat) under control. For Scull, psychiatry has been complicit in the implementation of a State-sponsored policy which resulted in the mentally ill (and other segregated groups) being decarcerated into an unprepared and unwelcoming community. The deinstitutionalisation of the mentally ill, argues Scull, is not the result of progressive developments in liberal-scientific psychiatry. Rather than the policy being driven by compassion (removing the mad from 'custodial warehouses' – i.e. the asylums) and the introduction of efficacious anti-psychotic drugs (not curing madness, but at least controlling symptoms), it has been economically determined. Scull argues that the reduction in the in-patient numbers commenced both in the USA and the UK either before or during the 1950s, whereas anti-psychotic drugs were only beginning to be used in the middle of the 1950s. Scull's point is that in the post-war period there was a fiscal crisis in the delivery of social policy whereby social control by segregation became too costly and therefore could not be justified.

Consequently, cheaper welfare options were sought, one of which was the programme of community care for the mentally ill. In part, Scull supports this position by suggesting that the former asylum inmates were not offered effective (and expensive) care in the community, but were neglected and ghettoised. Although Scull recognises that in Britain the pattern of decarceration has been to some degree different to that in the USA, the rise in the number of the mentally ill who are homeless, and who inhabit bed and breakfast accommodation, can be viewed as an example of the neglect and social exclusion of the mentally ill in the community (Morrall 1999).

However, Scull's approach can be criticised in a number of ways. For example, Busfield argues that with respect to the UK, Scull's account is defective on the basis of timing: 'The fiscal crisis of the state to which he refers is a phenomenon of the early 1970s and later, and not of the 1950s ...' (Busfield 1986: 329). Busfield suggests that, whilst Scull is correct to identify a 'mystification and distortion of a reality of neglect and lack of resources to those discharged from mental hospitals' (ibid.), he ignores the expansion of psychiatric services into primary health care.

Erich Fromm (1963) argues that it is (capitalist) society that is insane rather than individuals. Capitalism, for Fromm, is a form of social pathology. It contains major contradictions and irrationalities, that have immense social and economic consequences. For example, wars are fought regularly to protect markets. Periods of high unemployment alternate with periods of worker shortage. Mass entertainment, promulgated for profit, 'dumbs down' human activities, rendering life meaningless and devoid of interpersonal intimacy. An ethic of materialism, whereby commodities are valued above everything else, has replaced any semblance of spiritual or human-orientated regard of life.

Viviane Forrester describes the discrepancies in contemporary capitalism as engendering an 'economic horror'. Long-term unemployment in the West, where employment itself and the rules of work are now anachronistic, results in a kind of social hell for those who are marginalised:

> look for instance, at a luxurious, modern, sophisticated city, Paris, where so many people, the old or the new poor, sleep in the street, their bodies and minds wrecked by lack of nourishment, warmth, care, also togetherness and respect.
>
> (Forrester 1999: 28)

Using Fromm's and Forrester's analysis, madness can be seen to be the outcome of specific flaws in the social and economic fabric of society, not individual pathology. Humans degenerate physically and mentally because society is degenerative.

Thomas Szasz argues that mental disorder does not exist, and depicts the practice of psychiatry as illusionary, and the 'diseases' they deal with as ordinary (i.e. non medical) obstacles people have to cope with every day of their lives:

> It is customary to define psychiatry as a medical speciality concerned with the study, diagnosis, and treatment of mental illnesses. This is a worthless and misleading definition. Mental illness is a myth. Psychiatrists are not concerned with mental illnesses and their treatments. In actual practice they deal with personal, social, and ethical problems in living.
>
> (Szasz 1972: 269)

Szasz argues that psychiatry has persuaded the scientific community, the law, the media and the public that the effects of everyday human difficulties are really diseases (Szasz 1994). But for Szasz, much of what psychiatry deals with is not disease but 'behaviour'. These behaviours are related to problems with living, argues Szasz, and are not the province of medical science.

The social processes involved in the separation of 'normal' behaviour from 'abnormal' behaviour, however, are in themselves inconsistent and transient. For example, homosexuality, alcoholism, epilepsy and anorexia are all behaviours that have historically switched backwards and forwards from being embraced within tolerant notions of normality to being regarded as completely unacceptable. Moreover, a precise rendering of who has legitimacy over which form of misconduct is equally vaporous. Psychopathic behaviour and sexual abusiveness are two major areas of human misconduct that fall between legal and psychiatric categorisation.

Szasz also accuses psychiatry of projecting a fallacious correlation between 'diagnosis' and 'disease'. Diagnoses are fabricated epithets attributed to 'symptoms' or behaviours which may or may not correspond to actual disease entities. For Szasz, there is compatibility in the coupling of the diagnostic designation of 'malaria' with pathological alterations in the working of the human body, but there is no such synchronicity between psychiatric diagnostic labels and the 'illnesses' they purport to represent. This, argues Szasz, is why some psychiatric ailments (for example, masturbatory insanity) disappear from the medical textbooks. Mental diseases, states Szasz (1993), are not literalities but metaphors.

The forced confining in asylums and prisons of the mentally disordered, both in the past and at present, demonstrates for Szasz (1998) that although the 'illness' metaphor is used extensively, the social status of the mad is very different to that of the physically ill. The mentally disordered, argues Szasz, are treated in this way because they are assumed to have 'misbehaved' not because they are actually 'sick'.

The solution, however, for Szasz (1972), is the liberalisation of society along 'free-market' principles. The State and psychiatry should be stripped of their powers with respect to madness, and people should solve their problems with living by seeking redress from the law, or using private contracts with psychotherapists. Only those mental conditions that have an explicit organic causation should be treated by the profession of medicine.

For Foucault (1971), madness came to be viewed as placing in jeopardy the 'health' of 'rational' and social systems in a way that no other type of deviancy does. Madness intimidates those in authority so profusely because unintelligible actions and oratory, particularly if flaunted in the public arena, openly contest social norms based on sanity and reason.

Rationality was to become the essential ingredient of post-Enlightenment 'progress' towards a well-ordered civilisation, and the subsequent industrialisation of the Western world. The exposure of the population to flagrant 'nonsense' invalidates intellectual deduction, and scientific and technological invention. That is, the very credibility and perpetuity of the 'rationalist' paradigm is undermined by the 'crazed' behaviour and thoughts of the insane.

Mad thoughts and behaviours demonstrate a potential cultural counter-position for onlookers to adopt to that of rationalism. To think and behave differently is to offer a challenge to the dominant ideology, and may foster social unrest. Such unrest could lead to social change, which would displace those with 'rational' power.

Consequently, from Foucault's perspective, psychiatry protects society (and 'enjoys power' for itself in doing so – i.e. it is not operating purely on behalf of the State) by removing the unreasonable and irrational from a position of influence. This may be a literal removal from the public's sight to an asylum (where 'panoptic' observation can monitor the thoughts and behaviour of the mad). Other methods of restricting the influence of the mad might be through the use of chemicals (i.e. anti-psychotic drugs), or the 'therapeutic' readjustment of conduct and cognition.

Social disorganisation theorists argue that the organisation of cities produces such social problems as criminality and madness. Robert Faris and Warren Dunham (1965) suggest that the city can be broken down into a number of 'concentric-zones', whose characteristics either enhance 'normality' or boost deviancy. In their model of the city, the zone at the geographical centre is the commercial sector, containing shops, offices, small factories and places of entertainment. Today, this area may also be occupied by the homeless, within whose ranks the mentally disordered will be represented disproportionately (Craig *et al.* 1995). Those people without permanent residence take shelter in the nooks and crannies created by a bewildering display of architectural embellishment and anarchy typical of industrial and post-industrial design.

The next zone identified by Faris and Dunham is typified by slum housing, ghettos and rented accommodation. In this area reside various groups of new immigrants, the lower working class (semi-skilled and unskilled workers, many of whom are only partially employed), and sections of the 'underclass' (the permanently unemployed, criminal recidivists, drug users and dealers, and prostitutes). If and when the members of these groups are successful in terms of running businesses or finding employment, they have the opportunity to enter the third zone, which accommodates the 'stable working class' as well as former immigrants who are now more established within the social system.

In Britain, these last two zones have been 'gentrified' to some extent. That is, certain sections of the middle class (who are usually relatively young, either single or cohabiting, and without children) have 'converted' previously dilapidated housing into fashionable residences, thereby taking advantage of easy access to the centre of the city for work and entertainment.

Finally, situated on the edge of the city, there are the residential suburbs, the main habitation of the middle class. Today, however, there is also a growing minority of people who travel to the city from the countryside. Villages have seen the process of gentrification occur within their environs in the same way that it has occurred in the 'unfashionable' regions of the inner city.

Faris and Dunham argue that it is not the personalities and behaviour of the inhabitants that create the distinguishing features of these zones, it is the other way round. That is, it was evident that the environment dictated how people behaved as each location maintained its specific identity despite the movement of groups (for example Jewish immigrants being replaced by Hispanics in the USA, or Albanians succeeding North-Africans in Europe) through its parameters. Moreover, even though high rates of mobility occur within the most unstable area (found principally in the second zone, but also in the first and third zones), significant levels of officially recorded crime and deviance continue. In fact, the pace of population movement causes the anonymity and social isolation that then produce the conditions under which crime and deviancy (including mental disorders such as schizophrenia) will flourish.

Using labelling theory (from interactionist sociology), Thomas Scheff (1966) proposed that mental disorder was merely 'residual' rule-breaking. That is, when all other categories of deviance have been exhausted, then the label of 'madness' will be put to use by the agencies of social control (for example, the police, psychiatry and judges). This was particularly the case when the presentation of an 'unacceptable' behaviour is persistent, and has not attracted any other deviancy tag.

For Scheff, the remnant and lowly connotation of the label 'mad' was likely to stick to the individual permanently. Therefore, the mentally disordered person had little choice but to accept the proffered stereotype, and act accordingly. In Erving Goffman's (1963) terms, the individual who is stigmatised by a label such as mental disorder becomes socially discredited and discreditable, and has her or his identity 'spoiled' by the attitude of the 'normals'.

Stigma is explained by Goffman as any condition or attribute that draws towards it social condemnation and sanctions of one sort or another. He describes three different types of stigma, the first of which are 'abominations of the body' (a visible naevus or physical deformity). Second, are 'blemishes of individual character' (alcoholism, criminality, homosexuality, unemployment and mental disorder). Third, there is 'tribal stigma', whereby a group will be outcast on the basis of race, nationhood or religion.

Summary

There is a lot of madness about, but an agreed denotation remains illusive. It does not reflect credibly on medical science that there is so much confusion about what madness is, and that the history of medicine involves professional opportunism and barbaric procedures. However, the continued upsurge in developments in diagnostic techniques and treatment from the medical industries means that the understanding of madness as a genetic and/or biochemical malady is gaining strength.

The reputation of politicians, already tarnished beyond redemption, is further belittled as a consequence of the disordered policies towards the mad. But there does seem to be political will, albeit after centuries of State concern for madness, to have basic criteria for care.

Sociologists (and renegade psychiatrists) who promote the notion that madness does not exist (what is called madness being viewed as the product of a process of labelling, or the exercise of power), do little to help raise respect for their discipline. To deny that madness is, no matter in what cultural manifestation, an agonising and (usually) unwanted experience, is to be 'unreasonable'. To point out how social exclusion, stigma, bad habitation and materialism add to psychological suffering, is a far more realistic contribution to the debate over madness. To enhance the chances of mad people becoming 'citizens' with full human rights (Hazelton 1999), necessitates an acceptance of the reality of madness.

Further reading

Pilgrim, D. and Rogers, A. (1999) *A Sociology of Mental Health and Illness*, Buckingham: Open University Press, 2nd edn.

Chapter 10

Death

We are all going to die. All of our friends and family will also die. There is nothing so factual than the inevitability of our demise. Moreover, the predetermination of our death means that we are all in the process of dying. That is, dying is not something that happens only to those who will do so within a particular period of time.

Nurses wrestle with death throughout much of their working lives. They are part of an industry that has traditionally purported to have as its mission the alleviation of suffering and the preservation of life. They care for the dying, and help lay the dead to rest. However, on occasions the abatement of physical or emotional distress may actually lead to nurses and doctors killing their patients, either as a consequence of iatrogenesis, neglect or as a deliberate measure to end a patient's pain. The latter may involve (rarely) murder, the surreptitious removal of treatment or food, or the administration of types and dosages of medication that are known to induce death.

However, death is not all it seems. To begin with, some scientists (i.e. those persuaded by the logical positivism of Karl Popper 1959) may argue that not even death can be guaranteed. We may believe that people (as with all life forms) have always died. But, just as we cannot state categorically that the force of gravity, although it appears to have always worked in the past, will continue to make objects of any size drop to the ground at the same rate, death cannot be predicted (in the scientific sense) for everyone who is living now or who may be born in the future.

Moreover, the notion that death is certain for all living creatures depends on how 'life' and 'death' are defined, and who is doing the defining. That is, there is at times great ambiguity, both in terms of how the biological state of an organism is interpreted, and what social meaning is attached to that organism's condition.

Virtual death

Adults and children are exposed constantly to death. But, unlike previous epochs, where most people died in their homes and therefore were quite literally 'on display' to other members of their family, friends and neighbours, the expiration of life in the twenty-first century is experienced 'virtually'. Whilst death to some extent is a 'non-event' in modern society, barricaded as it is within the walls of hospitals, hospices and residential homes, it is conversely also a perennial and ubiquitous occupant of public space.

Throughout history, death has submitted itself nakedly as an everyday occurrence. People died at home, on the streets and whilst working. As Giddens (1997) notes, in pre-industrial society, many generations of a family lived in the same household. This is still the case (although it is becoming less common due to the effect of economic and cultural globalisation) for tribal communities in parts of Africa, Asia, South America and a number of South Sea Islands. Death happens as part of normal family life, and is much more firmly linked with the regeneration of life than is the case in industrial society. That is, in traditional cultures death is viewed as part of the 'life-cycle'. Moreover, death is not individualised to the same extent as in the West. The remains of the dead person are viewed as either materially or spiritually attached to those who are living. There is, therefore, an indefinite endurance of life.

In the agrarian and early industrial modes of production of the West, and in developing economic systems today, children have died young and in abundant numbers. Their 'overproduction' is testimony to the Grim Reaper's fondness for youth. However, the overproduction of children in these societies has caused and still causes the death of a significant number of women. Giving birth in the West was, and still is throughout the third world, a dangerous event.

Adults in ancient and feudal societies succumbed to death at half the average life-span for those now in the West. Moreover, most adults in the past did not die in old age (a category which in itself is unstable). Routine wars brought death to each village and town. But it was not until the First and Second World Wars, along with subsequent regional conflicts and civil strife, that such high percentages of the populace were annihilated. Since the twentieth century it has been possible to bring about the death of whole strata of society (for example, armies of young men; Jews; homosexuals; those Russians considered 'reactionary' by Joseph Stalin; the civilian populations of Hiroshima, Nagasaki and Dresden; Ibos tribes-people of Nigeria; Cambodians during the reign of the Khmer Rouge). The machinery and technology of war can produce death on a massive scale over a relatively short period of time, or (with nuclear weapons) instantaneously.

The effect on those who have been caught up in death during warfare can be devastating and socially divisive. Soldiers, despite training in killing, can not only suffer psychological damage as a consequence of causing the death of other humans, but may also find that on return from their fighting they are rejected by society. A common theme from American soldiers who had fought against the Viet Cong in the 1960s and 1970s was that they were marginalised by a society that wished to forget about such a military and political disaster. The fictional character of Agapeton Mandras in Louis de Bernières' novel *Captain Corelli's Mandolin*, an account of the defence of Greece from invasion by Italy and then Germany during the Second World War, expresses his realisation that seeing death in battle makes an individual feel 'different'. Mandras has come back dishevelled and distressed to his island home from the front line. Aware of the impact of the many deaths he has seen during the campaign against the fascist forces entering Greece from Albania, he ruminates about how his relationship with his mother and girlfriend has changed: 'There is a veil between me and them. ... I have been to war, and they have not; what do they know about anything?' (Bernières 1998: 140).

Most people in former times, however, died because of disease not warfare (or old age). In the past, epidemics of particular diseases brought death, which, in relative terms, killed more of the population than any war to date. The Black Death in England, which had spread from the Far East to Europe by plague-carrying fleas housed in the fur of rodents, wiped out perhaps 50 per cent of the population in 1348. Overall in Europe over a third of the population (25 million) died. In the 1350s and 1370s the plague struck again in Europe, devastating city-dwelling communities. Paris lost 50,000 of its citizens in 1437 to the *Yersinia Pestis* infection, the bacteria responsible for the plague. London (1665–66) and Vienna (1679) had further epidemics, which caused the deaths of up to 100,000 people in both cities. The plague continued to kill huge numbers in the eighteenth century (for example, in 1720, 48,000 died in Marseille, and in 1709, 300,000 died in Prussia).

Whilst the plague killed hundreds of thousands of people in India during the 1900s, and still poses a health risk in certain parts of Latin America and Africa, it has been controlled through the use of antibiotics. What the people of plague-infested cities had to suffer, however, during the Middle Ages was the brutish slaughter of loved ones, friends and neighbours, by a foe whose mode of conveying death was not recognised and/or managed effectively, thereby creating a further proliferation of deaths. Ironically, the killing of rats, rather than the offending fleas, resulted in more infection. A dead rat is of no use to a plague flea, so it will jump to the nearest and most numerous warm-blooded mammal ← humans. The scenes of decay and pain as (in the bubonic form of plague) the headaches increased in severity and the lymph nodes of the groin swelled enormously, or (in pneumonic plague) the lungs filled with pus and the coughing became severe and unstoppable, are hard to imagine. The bodies would then be transported through towns and villages by open cart to charnel-houses for burning. Therefore, no one, no matter what age or social standing, would escape the spectacle of death in its rawest and most barbaric form. Unless on a battlefield, where the entrails and limbs of fellow humans are torn from their bodies and strewn all around in a bloody blend of flesh and bones, there is no similar parade of tangible death in modern times.

Paradoxically, however, death is today readily available for our perusal and entertainment as a consistent theme in the content of radio, television and Internet news broadcasting. We may in the West, as Aries (1983) observed, be reticent to acknowledge death, talk about death, or admit to our own mortality, but death is no longer 'invisible'. Culturally, there remains a conversational 'taboo' with regard to the dying and death of those with whom we have an intimate relationship, and concerning our own necrotic fate as biological entities. However, the perishability of human corporeality is highly conspicuous in the 'information age'.

Death is exhibited starkly in documentaries on murders, wars and famine. Newspapers and popular magazines fill their columns with categorical details of homicides, suicides, accidents and obituaries. Visually and in narrative, the mass slaughter of men, women and children is reported recurrently throughout the media. The butchering of political and religious adversaries in Northern Ireland and Algeria, and the genocide in Bosnia and Rwanda, are delivered to a mass audience of death consumers. We gaze at the dead bodies being brought out of buckled trains in Germany, shattered aeroplane fuselages over South American mountains, and motorway pile-ups in Britain. We observe impotently and passively as the victims of drought in Somalia and floods in Mozambique, succumb to death.

We are treated to a steady diet of bloody mayhem not only in the media, but also in historical exposés of 'great tyrants' and imperial powers. In every high-street bookstore we can read elaborate accounts about, and view vivid photographs of, atrocities committed by the Nazis in Europe, the Americans in Vietnam, the British in India, the Japanese in China, Pol Pot in the Khmer Republic, or Saddam Hussein in Iraq.

The dissemination by the media of actual death, however, is supplemented by the omnipresence of fictional death. No radio, television, or theatre play (whether, drama, comedy or opera), or plot of a popular novel, is complete without a death (and sex) scene. Films and videos portray the gore of dying by gruesome means for a death-thirsty public. Children assassinate thousands of video-game and Internet-game combatants. Modern culture is saturated by the commercial manufacture of simulated death. Death has become, like sex, yet another commodity either in its own right or through which to sell other goods.

But these deaths are not experienced at first hand. The presentation and consumption of death, either in its real or artificial version, is mediated through the prism of electronic or documentary systems of communication. Death, therefore, has become both sanitised and 'hyperreal' (Baudrillard 1988). It belongs to a contrived realm of motion pictures and literature. Although we may see real death at some point in our lives, and will attend our own death, the countless numbers of other deaths we witness are experienced in a virtual world.

Social death

Death is a social occasion. By describing death in this way I do not simply mean that it is a time when people get together either to celebrate the life of the deceased or to mourn her or his death. What I am referring to is the manner in which society 'orchestrates' death.

For example, death is a social event in the sense that society produces the conditions under which people die, and loss of life is hastened. For example, every year thousands of people die through road accidents. Although it is improbable (unless merely in a tokenistic form), due to how unpopular such action would be, a government could bring in legislation concerning road safety that would slash the number of deaths caused by cars, lorries and other vehicles. Speed limits in cities could be reduced drastically; residential areas could be made traffic-free; all freight could be forced to go by rail; and exceptionally punitive fines and jail sentences could be introduced for speeding and drink-driving offences. It is not beyond the bounds of possibility that vehicle ownership could be banned completely, and the public left with public transport, bicycles, or walking to carry out their journeys. By not altering the circumstances that lead to the majority of fatalities on the roads, society is accepting that a large number of deaths (and consequent misery for the families of those who are killed) is the price paid for having a culture which values the freedom of movement by private vehicular transport, and an expeditious retail system.

The orchestration of death by society is also related to the issue of health inequalities. That is, the well-established relationship between social structure and mortality rates demonstrates that being poor, living in bad housing and being unemployed, will increase considerably your chances of dying younger than if you were materially well off and employed in a satisfying job.

Ivan Illich (1977) makes the point that the way death is conceptualised is related to the structures and beliefs of a society. Rituals, such as post-mortem examinations, coroners' reports, investigation by the police into 'suspicious deaths', mourning, wakes, cemetery dancing, the reading of a will, the making of a tombstone, burial in the ground, in a vesicle or pyre, and the satisfying of legal and financial obligations, are elements of the death event that are socially created. What rituals take place will differ from society to society.

Society's view on health will also affect how death is conceptualised. For Illich, the profession of medicine has intervened in life (by medicalising such personal or social conditions as pregnancy, illiteracy and madness), but is also responsible for refashioning death. Death has been expropriated by the medical profession. Doctors have successfully replaced purely religious connotations of death, which in themselves had supplanted pagan beliefs. Illich claims that the notion of a 'natural death', at the end of a 'healthy' life which is supposed to occur in old age, is a medicalised ideal which has at its core the image of the doctor struggling valiantly with potentially fatal ailments. If death happens at an earlier age, then it is considered 'untimely'. Medicine is striving continually to readjust the conditions under which death occurs, and at what age life ends. In this sense, all deaths today will be retrospectively reclassified as 'untimely'.

Moreover, Illich argues that the notion of death as a single God-given or normal event that is the same affair for everyone, has been reconfigured. Now there are multiple types of death, and an individual must be seen to have died from a specific condition. That is, people can die from one of a variety of forms of death, depending upon which fatal disease is diagnosed, and in which medical situation the death takes place. People now have to die of something – of one or more medical complaints. Moreover, they have to die somewhere – in a medical environment. This may be an intensive care unit, a medical or surgical ward, an accident and emergency room, operating theatre, a 'dying unit', or elderly care ward. If an individual dies in a hospice or residential home, or in their own home, she or he still attracts medical personnel and paraphernalia. The visiting general practitioner, district nurse, health-care assistant, disgorges the medical discourse even into the private bedroom of the dead. Dying on the roadside does not mean escape from the tentacles of the medical profession. An ambulance crew or mobile paramedics will be hailed, thereby signifying a medicalised death.

A classic study of the social organisation of dying and death within hospitals was conducted by Barney Glaser and Anselm Strauss (1965). The conclusions from the interactionist approach taken by these researchers still have application in today's health system. Glaser and Strauss produced a simple typology of communications which can be used to analyse more or less all health-care situations. Their model can reveal what forms of communication are transpiring between the key players in the drama of death. Such knowledge can enable patients and their significant others, and health-care practitioners, to produce overall and individual policies on what should or should not be divulged about the health status of the dying person.

The interactions between health personnel (principally doctors and nurses), relatives and the person who was dying were seen to fit into one of four *awareness contexts* in Glaser and Strauss' research. The first of these categories is *closed awareness*. Here the patient was not cognisant of her or his looming expiration. However others (i.e. the health practitioners and relatives) were. That is, the patient may understand that she or he is ill, and perhaps even realise that the illness is severe. But she or he does not comprehend fully that death rather than cure or living with a chronic condition is going to be the outcome.

The second context for Glaser and Strauss is that of *suspected awareness*. The patient surmises that others may know she or he is dying (and they do). Here both the patient and those around her or him are caught in a dilemma. For the patient, it may be better to have her or his suspicion confirmed or denied rather than being left in doubt. Hence, the patient may ask indirect questions to gain more clues, and these may be sought from people with whom she or he only has peripheral involvement, or who are junior members of the caring staff. Alternatively, the patient may bluntly ask her or his doctor, nurse or partner 'Am I going to die?'. For the staff caring for the dying patient and her or his relatives, the dilemma can be about whether or not to explain the reality of the situation if asked, or to give reassurance that this is not the case. Repudiating the patient's suspicions may be carried out in the belief that being aware of one's imminent death may hasten death.

Such preclusion, however, may also be the result of diagnostic uncertainty. That is, medical opinion may be less than absolute about the patient's condition and the chances of survival. Consequently, the verification of a patient's prospects as hopeless, and then to find that she or he has not died, may cause both professional embarrassment and possibly a lawsuit filed against the physician and/or the hospital. Furthermore, for some medical conditions (for example, AIDS), new medical treatments are constantly being found, and these may delay death beyond the expected point. A patient given a prognosis of only six months to live could find that a potent drug has been discovered during that period. The patient could then have the judgement of her or his life expectancy extended, and this may happen time and time again. In such circumstances, to tell a patient that death is assured would be inappropriate. Uncertainty here is not the result of medical-scientific fallibility, or communicative incompetence on behalf of health-care practitioners, but due to the vagaries of scientific invention.

If the patient takes the course of not seeking confirmation of her or his suspicions, then according to Glaser and Strauss a third context may be entered into, that of *mutual pretence awareness*. There is, they argue, a 'dying situation' in which everyone knows of the patient's condition, and the patient also understands that she or he has not long to live, but that all pretend that this is not the case. That is, there is an atmosphere of false hope generated from both the health-care staff and relatives, and the patient. No one admits candidly what all know to be the outcome of contracting the disease in question – death.

At variance with the other three contexts, *open awareness* occurs when all the relevant players (including the patient) acknowledge that the patient is dying. The subject of death, and the processes involved in dying, are discussed freely. This may take the form of the patient asking for information from health-care workers about what pain she or he might endure, talking over personal issues with her or his loved-ones, or making preparations for death (for example, settling financial matters). Of course, the patient may also become distraught, incapable of dealing with day-to-day activities such as eating and washing, let alone sorting out major issues such as wills and mortgages, and obsessed with the ephemerality of life. That is, it should not be assumed automatically that *open awareness* is synonymous with patient contentment.

In the situation of *closed awareness* there is not necessarily a deliberate attempt to 'protect' the dying person from knowing of her or his impending demise. Not telling the patient may be a way for the practitioners and relatives to avoid painful discussions on a subject that is not only distressing to them but for which they feel inadequately prepared. That is, practitioners and relatives may be safeguarding themselves from psychological anxiety, as a consequence of the 'taboo status' surrounding any talk about the real death of those near to us or our own death. A *closed awareness* context can therefore be viewed as not discrepant with the conventional social norms in the Anglo-Celtic cultures of the British Isles, Australasia and much of North America. Indeed, David Field (1989), who is in favour of more openness, nevertheless connects Western bio-medical treatments and medical practices to the practice of not telling patients about their ailments.

Moreover, the structural and cultural complexities of society may mean that to operate outside of this context can contravene accepted patterns of behaviour for certain ethnic minorities, age groups and social classes. It is also more likely to be the standard interactive pattern for men rather than women. Deborah Tannen's

(1992) description of stoicism, independence and achievement being male characteristics, and intimacy and sharing being female characteristics, suggests that the subject of dying may be more shut off from the former than the latter.

Furthermore, there is a tension between the social norms of either the dominant ideology of a society, or those adhered to by particular subdivisions of that society, and the practice of 'openness' advocated by many health-care professionals who care for the dying. This tension may be in part responsible for some of the ambiguity and apparent dishonesty that surround the contexts of *suspected awareness* and *mutual pretence awareness*.

For example, eminent writers in the field of dying, such as Kubler-Ross (1969), have attacked Western society as 'death-defying'. They have portrayed the dying person, on discovering that she or he has a fatal disease, as undergoing a number of emotional stages. For Kubler-Ross, this begins with *denial* whereby the patient refuses to believe that she or he is really going to die. Second, there is *anger*. At this stage the patient is resentful about dying, questioning why she or he has been chosen to die, and may become hostile towards those who are delivering care or relatives and friends. According to Kubler-Ross, the third stage is one of *bargaining*. Here the patient attempts to negotiate with those (for example, her or his doctor, or God) they consider have the power to 'reinterpret' or reverse their advance towards death. In the next stage, denial of, anger about, and bargaining over dying is replaced by a feeling of *depression*. Finally, there is *acceptance*, with the patient becoming calmer and preparing herself or himself to let go of life.

Within this multi-staged psychological framework of dying, there is an assumption that the acceptance of death is more healthy for the patient than remaining in denial or continuing to execute rage. There is also an apparent perpetration of an open awareness (at least on behalf of the health-care practitioners and relatives) mode of communication in all of the stages. However, such a policy concerning dying is culturally naive. Not only is there evidence that the stages of dying set out by Kubler-Ross cannot be generalised, but no such scheme can possibly fit all the variants associated with human behaviour and emotions, nor the multitude of cultural differences that exist within the West (Young and Cullen 1996).

Moreover, not addressing the complex effects of social structure and cultural diversity on individual behaviour is only part of the criticism that can be levelled at a policy of blanket openness. By arguing that more notice should be taken of how other societies and cultures cope with dying and death, there is the assumption that the customs of the West are faulty. Hence Kubler-Ross and her followers are reproducing the essential paradox of the cultural relativist argument. There is an unfeasible leap of logic from wanting to pay homage to the 'rightfulness' of a number of (non-Western) cultures whilst criticising the 'wrongfulness' of other (Western) cultures. Put simply, what the 'correct' conduct for a doctor, nurse, relative and patient from New York, Edinburgh, or Melbourne should be in the dying process, cannot be extracted from observing what social scripts are followed when an Inuit, Fijian or Peruvian Indian is dying. This is reverse cultural imperialism. It is not the West that is (as is more usual) exporting its values to non-industrial or developing societies, but the values of the latter that are being imported to the West.

Indeed it has been argued in a study by McIntosh (1977) that most of the patients he interviewed who were dying, although they knew they were extremely ill, did not want to know the actual diagnosis and prognosis for fear of discovering that they were going to die. Many of these patients, according to McIntosh, put forward questions, and interpreted the information they were given, in such a way as to have only 'good' news about their condition. For health-care practitioners to engender an 'open' dialogue, therefore, would be both difficult and disrespectful of the patient's apparent wish to remain deluded. However, in McIntosh's study the patients' convoluted communications with medical staff were complicated further by the discrepancy between the overt and subliminal messages being given by doctors. Although the doctors stated that they would provide the patients with the facts regarding their illness, they were apparently reluctant to do so without a good deal of prompting.

Furthermore, Tony Walter (1991), examining the situation in Britain, has argued that the notion of death being 'taboo' needs to be reassessed. He suggests that since the 1960s a more 'expressive' culture has developed, certainly amongst the middle classes, which makes it more possible to talk about death. However, the reduction of death rates in modern society means that 'real' death does not occur as often, or when it does it happens out of sight within institutions. Moreover, most people die today when they are elderly, rather than in the past when death was much more common amongst those in the 'prime of life'. Previously, death was not only happening more frequently, but loss was experienced more intensely. The adults who died were important, if not essential, to the economy and emotional stability of their families. For Walter, therefore, it is hardly surprising that in the modern world people appear not to be competent at handling bereavement on a personal level, or that modern society does not possess meaningful ritualistic modes of expression in comparison with pre-modern societies. People today in the West are not 'denying' death. They have little opportunity to 'avow' death. Society, therefore, has barely any requirement for intricate and communal death liturgies.

A further study by Glaser and Strauss (1968) can also be considered classic in the re-conceptualisation of death and dying away from being understood merely as natural processes, and towards acknowledging their social significance. From their observations of dying in hospitals, Glaser and Strauss suggested that people who were dying went through various social phases, which they described as *critical junctures*. These junctures, which refer to the socially organised process of dying, are not to be confused with the psychological stages as denoted by, for example, Kubler-Ross. The difference is that Glaser and Strauss, rather than focusing mainly on the internal mechanisms of the dying person, were cognisant of the socio-environmental factors in the vicinity of a projected death and the effect of these factors on the patient's social status. For Glaser and Strauss the patient who is dying undertakes a certain 'career-pathway' from the point of the announcement of her or his terminal state to when death occurs. What should happen at each part of the dying career of the patient, and how long the careers should last, is decreed by the expectations and reactions of the doctors and nurses who have responsibility for the patient, but who also have to take into account other administrative and organisational regulations and obligations. That is, the trajectory of the patient's dying career is mapped out by the doctors and nurses on the basis of what they believe to be the normal pattern for people with similar complaints. However, the bureaucratic design of the hospital will impinge on how the dying career of the patient is managed.

The ward staff may assume that a patient suffering from, for example, inoperable cancer of the stomach, with untreatable cancerous metastases in other organs, and who is irreversibly emaciated, will die within a few weeks. Local health-care resources (which themselves are affected by health policies at a national level), will be formulated on the basis of how much care can be allocated to this patient, and similar patients. Staff shifts and numbers are arranged, and clinical equipment and palliative therapies ordered, in an attempt to satisfy both the immediate needs of this patient and a generalised programme of care for others with equivalent diseases. Care is controlled, therefore, by financial considerations and organisational norms, as well as by clinical decisions.

There are commonly, suggest Glaser and Strauss, seven *critical junctures*. The first commences when the patient is defined as dying by the clinical staff. She or he is reclassified (perhaps not knowing if a *closed awareness* context is operating) from either a 'healthy person' or a 'patient' (i.e. a person with an illness) to a person who is 'dying'. Consequently, there is a dramatic loss of social standing as the label of 'dying' signifies a path towards being a person for whom there is no hope and no future. There is, therefore, a 'non-person' social ranking awaiting that individual as death approaches.

Michael Young and Lesley Cullen (1996) examined the meanings fourteen patients (who had only months to live) and their carers attached to their respective lives following the diagnosis of cancer. Cancer, unlike for example, death from a heart attack, represents a 'slow death'. Incidents of 'slow death' in the West are increasing given the greater numbers of people dying from cancer compared to 'quick deaths' from infectious diseases, accidents or wars. There is, therefore, with cancer a much greater chance of depersonalisation because dying is prolonged, but also because of the recognised severity of the disease:

> people quite suddenly stopped being people and became pa-tients under someone else's orders. It was not for nothing that people customarily spoke of being 'under' – 'I am under the doctor'. … They could cease overnight to be a person – or at any rate the same person when they were consigned to wait in giant buildings (the largest buildings many people go into) full of bustling strangers in white coats who, though strangers, may well have a terrifying power of clairvoyance about their future.
>
> (Young and Cullen 1996: 38)

The second *critical juncture* happens when the relatives and friends of the dying person start to make emotional and practical preparations for the death. If the patient realises that she or he is going to die (particularly if there is an *open awareness* context), then she or he may also adjust emotionally to the situation. Following this, there will be, in the third *critical juncture*, what Glaser and Strauss describe as the 'nothing more to do' phase. That is, there has been a diagnosis and preparations for death have been made, but the individual concerned has not yet reached the steeply descending part of the death career. There is, therefore a lull in proceedings (practical and emotional) with loved ones not knowing how comforting to be to the dying person. Nursing staff may handle this period before the plunge towards death by avoiding close contact with the patient. It is at this point that the depersonalisation of the patient may become transparent.

The next four junctures involve overlapping phases which collectively make up the concluding interval of life. Lasting many hours or several days, the fourth *critical juncture* is classified as the 'final descent'. The routine on the hospital ward will alter noticeably. For example, the patient may be placed in a side-room and nursed more intensively. Extra pain-killing drugs or higher dosages may be prescribed. Visiting hours may be extended, with perhaps many more relatives and friends making an appearance. The fifth *critical juncture* heralds in the 'last hours' during which last rights may be administered or other religious ceremonies conducted. This is followed by the sixth *critical juncture*, the 'death watch'. Here a partner or near relative may choose to be with the dying person all day and night, or a nurse may be assigned to provide exclusive care and company.

Finally comes the death. Apart from being the catalyst for a number of cultural rituals depending upon the dead person's faith (or lack of it), the death invokes all manner of organisational formalities: the medical sanctification of death; the reclassifying of the person from 'the patient' to 'the deceased'; the cleansing of the body; wrapping the body in a shroud; transfer of the body to the mortuary; the washing-down of the (ex)patient's bed and removal of 'its' belongings; the registering of the event in the nurses and doctors records; informing the coroner.

So, the scene is pre-set for the patient to play her or his social role in the institutionalised drama of dying. All a dying patient has to do is to follow the designated trajectory towards death. This drama, however, is somewhat exceptional. Unlike most plays, the central character (and some of the supporting actors – i.e. the relatives) have not been given a copy of the script. That is, the patient is generally unaware that a trajectory for her or his death has been formulated, and that her or his fate is being 'organised'. Where the foreseen trajectory is not followed, and given the clandestine nature of its existence it is highly possible that this will be a frequent occurrence, there will be much consternation for both the relatives and the hospital staff. If, for example, the final descent is delayed (i.e. there is a slower trajectory than predicted) or sudden (i.e. there is a quicker trajectory than anticipated), then it may wreck the emotional strategies of the loved ones, and cause havoc to the administrative plans of the ward staff. Patients are expected, therefore, to die within their allotted trajectory 'with good grace' and to have a 'good death'.

Inequitable death

David Sudnow (1967), like Glaser and Strauss, has made a major contribution to the sociological study of death. His observations of the interactions between nursing and medical staff and their 'dead' patients in the emergency ward of a public hospital in the USA have illustrated how, depending on the condition and inferred social status of the patient, deaths are dealt with very differently.

That is, there is a 'social inequality' in death and dying. Judgements are made by doctors and nurses about the prestige and character of a patient, with much more effort being made to revive those who are perceived to be young or wealthy, and much less effort delivered to those considered to be old or morally repugnant. The older a person is, the poorer she or he is considered to be, and the more socially undesirable, the quicker the pronouncement of death.

For example, Sudnow noticed that there was a dramatic eleven-hour-long attempt by doctors and nurses to revive a young child who was brought into the emergency ward with the standard 'signs of death' (i.e. no detectable heartbeat or breathing). However, the arrival of an elderly woman in the emergency ward with the same signs of death resulted in no medical intervention whatsoever, except that she was immediately pronounced dead.

In Sudnow's study, people who were regarded as alcoholics, 'dope' addicts, prostitutes, violent, vagrants and those who had apparently committed suicide, were generally declared dead relatively quickly. For Sudnow, however, any patient (dead or alive) who attends a public hospital in the USA is already denoted as socially 'inferior' compared to those who receive the services of private health care.

Akin to Glaser and Strauss' (1968) idea that dying people are depersonalised, Sudnow argued that a distinction can be drawn between 'biological' death and 'social' death. That is, Sudnow suggested that the hospital staff in his study regarded some patients who were not 'clinically' dead (i.e. the 'signs of life' – breathing and a palpable pulse – were still apparent), as corpses.

However, the reverse may also be true. Patients who die biologically (where there is a complete cessation of the bodies' organic functioning) may still be regarded as being 'alive' in that relatives may not accept that their loved one has died (Mulkay 1993). The biologically dead person may be talked to, or thought about, by her or his relatives as if the death had not occurred. Referring to the dead as though they are alive may either be short-lived (for example, the actuality of death may be affirmed by the attitude of hospital staff and the burial procedures), or long-term (for example, a lost child or partner may considered to be surviving 'spiritually', embodied within an inanimate object).

Sudnow also commented on how people termed 'DOAs' (dead on arrival) are dealt with. Ambulance staff were instructed to refer to people they suspected of being dead as 'possible' DOAs because only a physician could certify a 'sure' death. This procedure is demanded by the hospital authorities for legal and (in the USA) insurance purposes. Therefore, a person who is dead cannot be described as such until a doctor provides confirmation of that state. What then is the status of that person prior to the doctor's confirmation of death? Is she or he 'alive', or in an ontological void whereby she or he is neither living nor deceased?

In an update of Sudnow's work, Stefan Timmermans (1998) conducted a study of two USA hospitals in which he observed 112 scenes of resuscitation, and interviewed forty-two health-care practitioners including doctors, nurses, social workers and chaplains. As Timmermans points out, the management of health care and medical science has changed dramatically since Sudnow's research in the 1960s. In particular, resuscitation theories, techniques and equipment have been overhauled, and hospitals have installed formal 'protocols' indicating the correct procedures that should be followed by medical and nursing staff.

Paradoxically, argues Timmermans, these developments in medical science, and formalisation of practices, have served merely to justify decisions made by hospital staff about who to resuscitate, and how much effort should be made to preserve life. Timmermans concludes that changes in health-care practice have not substantially altered the appropriateness of Sudnow's concept of social inequalities in death. For example, age remains a major factor in determining the social viability of a patient. Moreover, if the health-care workers involved in the resuscitation process identified the patient as a 'drunk' or 'drug abuser' then less effort would be made. Aggressive use of the instruments of revival, and implementation of medical protocols, is preserved for those who are either known to those working in emergency wards, or who are perceived to have similar or higher cultural attributes. For the socially substandard, equipment and protocols are utilised 'ritualistically'.

Summary

Society is ambiguous towards death. Some deaths are encouraged blatantly. Huge numbers of people are killed in times of war. In times of peace, significant numbers of people are allowed to die as a consequence of transport and health policies, and the need to keep shops full of fashionable commodities.

Moreover, whilst 'real' death is kept concealed, 'virtual' death is flaunted. Death is a perpetual feature of news broadcasting and popular entertainment.

There is also ambiguity with respect to when a person can be classified as 'dying' and 'dead'. Both death and dying have become medical categories rather than natural events, and are affected by the contexts, junctures, and biases of the health-care system.

Further reading

Taylor, M. and Cullen, L. (1996) *A Good Death*, London: Routledge.

Conclusion

In this book I have applied the 'imagination' of sociology to health-care issues that have relevance to nursing work. The purpose of such an appraisal is to engender 'thinking'. It is also to give direction to the practical aspects of nursing work.

Sociological thinking and pragmatism stem from the application of theoretical perspectives to social and natural events. Through such a process, events are laid bare (or at least more undressed than they would otherwise be), and can thereby have their worth and characteristics inspected more accurately.

Three themes can be identified in the material presented in the book. These are: conceptual ambiguity; authoritative deception; sociological cynicism.

Ambiguity

There is an imprecision about the common concepts that nurses, their clinical colleagues, and policy makers utilise in the business of delivering health care. It is astounding to realise that the health policies of governments, supra-national health agencies, and organisations representing health-care practitioners and health-care consumers base their strategies and resource priorities on vague and conflicting understandings of the essence of their industry – 'health' and 'illness'. We simply cannot say that when patients, practitioners and politicians use these terms that they are referring to the same phenomena. That is, being 'ill' (the subjective experience of somatic and/or psychological malfunction) is not concordant with having a 'disease' (the medical consigning of a diagnosis).

Moreover, the state of 'sickness' indicates the existence of a social role. Being sick encompasses both illness and disease, and the imposition of social rights and obligations. Consequently, what has to be acknowledged is that society as well as biology has a major impact on health, and that people must be consulted about what they believe is health and what treatments they wish to have. That is, social factors and personal understandings have to be part of the overall mapping of health and illness.

Sex, madness and death are also poorly conceived by health practitioners. Given that these entities are so integral to humanity, and that they permeate society (both in their material and virtual forms) there is an astonishing degree of uncertainty about what they are and how they should be handled. Moreover, sexual disease, madness and death, have biological antecedents, but are influenced by social and organisational norms.

Deception

Power-games are enacted by the elites in society and by the various occupational groups that are involved in health care. The brandishing of power by the State coerces those considered 'deviant' (including the 'sick') into performances intended to limit social instability. The wielding of power by health-care practitioners regulates how much control those with illness can have over their treatment. The empowerment of the patient, therefore, is only possible if the State and its agencies of control relinquish their power.

Professional power has also been responsible for manipulating the population in general into accepting that the experience of living rests upon (indefinite) medical and health beliefs. Furthermore, occupational groups such as medicine have flourished by using their power to gain freedom of action in their work, and to eclipse other contenders from the same field.

The profession of medicine has basked in the epistemological grandeur of science. However, whilst science can and does offer a discerning perception of the world that has aided human and medical development tangibly, social processes direct which subjects are to be studied, by whom and for what purpose. That is, both medicine and science provide answers to human problems that no other explanatory framework can match, but neither should be considered to inhabit an epistemological plane untainted by cultural values and personal motivations.

However, the most mendacious game is that of instructing individuals to become more healthy when a major contributor to ill-health is social inequality. People need to stop smoking, avoid harmful food and exercise more habitually. But society also needs to reform its structures and surroundings by providing better housing, meaningful employment, adequate wages, improved working conditions, efficient transport systems and an unpolluted environment.

Cynicism

Scepticism abounds in sociology. Whatever subject sociologists tackle, whether this be education, criminal justice, politics, the media or health care, there will inevitably be the supposition that exploitation and misrepresentation are present. This is just the nature of the beast. To have the imagination to see that, behind the front-stage of human action and the façade of social institutions, there are intentions, processes and structures, that manipulate and refashion the underlying 'facts', leads to the suspicion that everything is false and everyone is biased.

The explication presented in this book, however, has not just been critical of the concepts and practices that underpin health care, and the covert use of power by the State and dominant groups (especially medicine). These are traditional remits of sociological analysis in this area.

What I have also taken umbrage at is the type of sociology that is instinctively antagonistic to medical and (less often) nursing practice, and science, and proclaims that illnesses are social fabrications. Sociologists, scientists, doctors and nurses have a moral responsibility to collate their intellectual skills and bodies of knowledge, and donate to the problem of world suffering imaginative solutions that are not hidebound by interdisciplinary warfare and infinitely regressive conceptual deconstruction.

Appendix

Practice grid

Theory (identify the specific theory/perspective)	Principles (list the main principles of theory)	Implications for practice (apply the theory to YOUR practice – list insights gained and changes that can be made)

References

Abbott, P. and Wallace, C. (eds) (1990) *The Sociology of the Caring Professions*, London: Falmer Press.

Abraham, J. (1995) *Science, Politics and the Pharmaceutical Industry*, London: University College London Press.

Aggleton, P. (1990) *Health*, 1st edn, London: Routledge.

Allan, G. (ed.) (1999) *The Sociology of the Family*, Oxford: Blackwell.

Andrews, J., Porter, R., Tucker, P. and Waddington, K. (1997) *The History of Bethlem*, London: Routledge.

Aries, P. (1983) *The Hour of Our Death*, Harmondsworth: Penguin.

Armstrong, D. (1984) 'The patient's view', *Social Science and Medicine*, 18 (9), 737–44.

Baker, R. (1996) *Sperm Wars: Infidelity, Sexual Conflict, and Other Bedroom Battles*, London: Fourth Estate.

Baran, P. (1973) *The Political Economy of Growth*, Harmondsworth: Penguin.

Baudrillard, J. (1988) *Selected Writings*, Stanford, CA: Stanford University Press.

Beck, U. (1992) *Risk Society: Towards a New Modernity*, trans. M. Ritter, London: Sage.

Becker, H.S. (1963) *Outsiders: Studies in the Sociology of Deviance*, Glencoe: Free Press.

Bell, D. (1973) *The Coming of the Post-Industrial Society*, New York: Basic Books.

Bennett, C. (1998) 'In the blood or in the head?', *Guardian*, 1 June.

Berger, P. and Luckman, T. (1967) *The Social Construction of Reality: A Treatise in the Sociology of Knowledge*, Harmondsworth: Penguin.

Bernières, L. de (1998) *Captain Corelli's Mandolin*, London: Vintage.

Bhaskar, R. (1998) 'Philosophy and scientific realism', in M. Archer, R. Bhaskar, A. Collier, T. Lawson and A. Norrie (eds), *Critical Realism: Essential Readings*, London: Routledge, chap. 1, pp. 16–47.

Blair, T. (1999) 'Foreword' by the Prime Minister to *Saving Lives: Our Healthier Nation*, London: Department of Health, Stationery Office.

Blane, D. (1999) 'The life course, the social gradient, and health', in M. Marmot and R.G. Wilkinson (eds), *Social Determinants of Health*, Oxford: Oxford University Press, chap. 4, pp. 64–80.

Blaxter, M. (1990) *Health and Lifestyles*, London: Tavistock.

Bocock, R. (1976) *Freud and Modern Society*, London: Van Nostrand Reinhold.

Borger, J. (1999) 'US bid to own gene rights', *Guardian*, 25 October.

Boseley, S. (1998a) 'The doctors' dilemma', *Guardian*, 13 May.

—— (1998b) 'Medical studies "rubbish" ', *Guardian*, 24 June.

—— (1999a) 'Trial and error puts patients at risk', *Guardian*, 27 July.

—— (1999b) 'Mail order aids fail to win clean bill of health', *Guardian*, 7 December.

—— (2000) ' "Flying doctors" investigate', *Guardian*, 28 January.

Bradbury, M. (1975) *The History Man*, London: Secker and Warburg.

Brindle, D. (1997) 'Defence budget dwarfed by £32 billion mental health bill', *Guardian*, 10 October.

—— (2000) 'Doctors say "vague" GMC is failing them', *Guardian*, 3 March.

Brooks, P. (1993) *Body Works: Objects of Desire in Modern Narrative*, Cambridge, MA: Harvard University Press.

Browne, A. (1999) 'Tough new warnings raise the heat on the war on smoking', *Observer*, 14 November.

Brundtland, G.H. (2000) *Health and Population*, BBC Reith Lectures 2000, London: BBC.

Brunner, E. and Marmot, M. (1999) 'Social organisation, stress, and health', in M. Marmot and R.G. Wilkinson (eds), *Social Determinants of Health*, Oxford: Oxford University Press, chap. 2, pp. 17–43.

Burne, J. (2000) 'Healing in harmony', *Guardian Weekend*, 26 February.

Burrows, R., Nettleton, S. and Bunton, R. (1995) 'Sociology and health promotion: health, risk and consumption under late modernism', in R. Bunton, S. Nettleton and R. Burrows (eds), *The Sociology of Health Promotion*, London: Routledge, chap. 1, pp. 1–9.

Busfield, J. (1986) *Managing Madness: Changing Ideas and Practice*, London: Unwin Hyman.

Buss, D.M. (1994) *The Evolution of Desire*, New York: Basic Books.

Carr-Saunders, A.M. and Wilson, P.A. (1933) *The Professions*, Oxford: Clarendon Press.

Carter, H. (1999) 'Anger as model's eggs go on sale', *Guardian*, 10 October.

Cartner-Morley, J. (1998) 'Doctors in disgrace: one month's headlines', *Guardian*, 22 October.

Carvel, J. (1998) 'Citizenship may enter curriculum', *Guardian*, 1 May.

Christie, I. (1999) 'Return of sociology', *Prospect*, January (Internet highlights: http://www.prospect-magazine.co.uk), 1–5.

Clarke, L. (1999) 'Nursing in search of a science: the rise and rise of the new nurse brutalism', *Mental Health Care*, 2 (8), 270–2.

Cockerham, W.C. (1996) *Sociology of Mental Disorder*, Upper Saddle River, NJ: Prentice Hall, 4th edn.

Collee, J. (1995) Untitled, *Observer Magazine*, 15 January.

Collins, B.E. and Raven, B.H. (1969) 'Group structure: attraction, coalitions, communications and power', in G. Lindzey and E. Aronson (eds), *The Handbook of Social Psychology*, vol. 4, 2nd edn, Reading, MA: Addison-Wesley, chap. 30, pp. 102–204.

Comte, A. (1853) *The Positive Philosophy*, trans. M. Martineau, London: Trubner.

Connell, R.W. (1996) *Masculinities*, Cambridge: Polity.

Conrad, P. and Schneider, J.W. (1980) *Deviance and Medicalisation: From Badness to Sickness*, St Louis, MI: Mosby.

Consumers' Association (1999) 'Management of tension-type headache', *Drug and Therapeutics Bulletin*, 37 (6), 41–4.

Coppock, V. and Hopton, J. (2000) *Critical Perspectives on Mental Health*, London: Routledge.

Craig, T., Bayliss, E., Klein, O., Manning, P. and Reader, L. (1995) *The Homeless Mentally Ill Initiative: An Evaluation of Four Clinical Teams*, London: Department of Health/Mental Health Foundation.

Crawford, R. (1980) 'Healthism and the medicalisation of everyday life', *International Journal of Health Services*, 10 (3), 365–83.

Crook, S., Pakulski, J. and Waters, M. (1992) *Postmodernization: Change in Advanced Society*, London: Sage.

Darwin, C. (1998, original 1859) *The Origin of Species*, Oxford: Oxford World's Classics, 1998.

Davey, B. and Seale, C. (eds) (1996) *Experiencing and Explaining Disease*, Buckingham: Open University Press.

Davies, J.K. and Macdonald, G. (1998) *Quality, Evidence, and Effectiveness in Health Promotion: Striving for Certainties*, London: Routledge.

Dawkins, R. (1994) 'Science's social standing: the moon is not a calabash', *The Times Higher Education Supplement*, 30 September.

Department of Health (1992) *The Health of the Nation: A Strategy for Health in England*, London: Department of Health.

—— (1997) *The New National Health Service: Modern, Dependable*, London: Stationery Office.

—— (1998a) *Government Committed to Public Health Crusade Against Inequalities – Dobson* (Press release 98/298), London: Department of Health.

—— (1998b) *National Confidential Inquiry into Perioperative Deaths*, London: Department of Health.

—— (1998c) *The New National Health Service*, White Paper, London: Stationery Office.

—— (1999a) *Commission For Health Improvement* (press release, 1999/0558), London: Department of Health.

—— (1999b) *Saving Lives: Our Healthier Nation*, Department of Health. London: Stationery Office.

—— (2000a) *National Health Service Plan: A Plan for Investment, A Plan for Reform*, London: Stationery Office.

—— (2000b) *Revolution in Casualty Care* (press release 2000/118), London: Department of Health.

Delanty, G. (1997) *Social Science: Beyond Constructivism and Realism*, Buckingham: Open University Press.

Dingwall, R. (1986) 'Anatomy of a profession: training for a varied career', *Nursing Times*, 82 (13), 27–8.

Dobson, R. (1998) 'Kill or cure', *Guardian*, 29 September.

Douglas, J. (1996) 'Developing with black and minority ethnic communities, health promotion strategies which address social inequalities', in P. Bywaters and E. McLeod (eds), *Working for Equality in Health*, London: Routledge, chap. 12, pp. 179–96.

Dubos, R. (1959) *Mirage of Health: Utopias, Progress and Biological Change*, New York: Harper and Row.

Durham, M. (1998) 'Doctors treat distant patients via video link', *Observer*, 7 June.

Durkheim, E. (1897) *Suicide*, New York: Free Press, 1966

—— (1957) *Professional Ethics and Civic Morals*, London: Routledge and Kegan Paul.

Eden, R. (2000) 'Abolish the GMC "to protect patients" ', *Daily Telegraph*, 7 June.

Emmel, N.D. and D'Souza, L. (1999) 'Health effects of forced evictions in the slums of Mumbai', *The Lancet*, 354, 25 September, 1118.

Engels, F. (1892) *The Condition of the Working Class in England*, St Albans: Granada.

Etzioni, A. (ed.) (1998) *The Essential Communitarian Reader*, Lanham, MD: Rowman and Littlefield.

Evans-Pritchard, E.E. (1937) *Witchcraft, Oracles and Magic among the Azande*, Oxford: Clarendon.

Faris, R. and Dunham, W. (1965) *Mental Disorders in Urban Areas*, Chicago, IL: University of Chicago Press.

Featherstone, M., Hepworth, M. and Turner, B. (1991) *The Body: Social Processes and Cultural Theory*, London: Sage.

Fennell, P. (1996) *Treatment without Consent: Law, Psychiatry and the Treatment of Mentally Disordered People since 1845*, London: Routledge.

Feyerabend, P. (1975) *Against Method*, London: New Left Books.

Field, D. (1989) *Nursing the Dying*, London: Tavistock/Routledge.

Fletcher, R. (1962) *Britain in the Sixties: The Family and Marriage*, Harmondsworth: Penguin.

Forrester, V. (1999) *The Economic Horror*, Cambridge: Policy.

Foucault, M. (1967) *Madness and Civilisation – A History of Insanity in the Age of Reason*, London: Tavistock.

—— (1971) *Madness and Civilisation*, London: Tavistock.

—— (1973) *The Birth of the Clinic: An Archaeology of Medical Perception*, New York: Pantheon.

—— (1985) *The Use of Pleasure: The History of Sexuality*, vol. 2, Harmondsworth: Penguin.

Fox, N. (1992) *The Social Meaning of Surgery*, Buckingham: Open University Press.

Freidson, E. (1970a) *The Profession of Medicine: A Study of the Applied Sociology of Knowledge*, New York: Dodd Mead.

—— (1970b) *Professional Dominance: The Social Structure of Medical Care*, Chicago: Atherton Press.

—— (1988) *The Profession of Medicine: A Study of the Applied Sociology of Knowledge – With a New Afterword*, Chicago, IL: University of Chicago Press.

—— (1994) *Professionalism Reborn: Theory, Prophecy and Policy*, Cambridge: Polity Press.

French, J. and Raven, B. (1953) 'The bases of social power', in D. Cartwright and A. Zander (eds), *Group Dynamics*, London: Tavistock, pp. 259–69.

Freud, S. (1930) 'Civilisation and its discontents', in J. Strachey (ed.), *The Standard Edition of the Complete Works of Sigmund Freud*, vol. XXI, London: Hogarth.

Friday, N. (1976) *My Secret Garden: Women's Sexual Fantasies*, London: Quartet Books.

—— (1991) *Women on Top: How Real Life Has Changed Women's Sexual Fantasies*, London: Hutchinson.

Fromm, E. (1963) *The Sane Society*, London: Routledge and Kegan Paul.

Gamarnikow, E. (1978) 'Sexual division of labour: the case of nursing', in A. Kuhn and A. Wolpe (eds), *Feminism and Materialism: Women and their Modes of Production*, London: Routledge and Kegan Paul, pp. 96–123.

Geary, R. (1998) *Essential Criminal Law*, London: Cavendish, 2nd edn.

Gibson, C.H. (1991) 'A concept analysis of empowerment', *Journal of Advanced Nursing*, 16, 354–61.

Giddens, A. (1991) *Modernity and Self-identity: Self and Society in the Late Modern Age*, Cambridge: Polity Press.

—— (1997) *Sociology*, Cambridge: Polity, 3rd edn.

—— (1998) *The Third Way: The Renewal of Social Democracy*, Cambridge: Polity.

—— (1999) Runaway World: Lecture 2, BBC Reith Lectures, Internet site: http://news.bbc.co.uk/hi/english/static/events/reith_99/week2.html, pp. 1–6.

Gittins, D. (1998) *Madness in its Place: Narratives of Severalls Hospital*, London: Routledge.

Glaser, B. and Strauss, A. (1965) *Awareness of Dying*, Chicago, IL: Aldine.

—— (1968) *Time for Dying*, Chicago, IL: Aldine.

Goffman, E. (1961) *Asylums*, Harmondsworth: Penguin.

—— (1963) *Stigma: Notes on the Management of Spoiled Identity*, Harmondsworth: Penguin.

Gomm, R. (1996) 'Mental health and inequality', in T. Heller, J. Reynolds, R. Gomm, R. Mustan and S. Pattison (eds), *Mental Health Matters: A Reader*, Basingstoke: Macmillan/Open University Press, chap. 14, pp. 110–20.

Goodwin, S. (1997) *Comparative Mental Health Policy*, Sage: London.

Gotzshe, P. and Olsen, O. (2000) 'Is screening for breast cancer with mammography justifiable?', *The Lancet*, 335 (9198), 129–34.

Hardyment, C. (1998) 'We are family', *Prospect*, June, 36–9.

Haug, M. (1973) 'De-professionalisation: an alternative hypothesis for the future', in P. Halmos (ed.), *Professionalisation and Social Change*, Sociological Review Monograph 20, Keele: University of Keele.

Hazelton, M. (1999) 'Mental health and citizenship', in C. Grbich (ed.), *Health in Australia: Sociological Concepts and Issues*, Sydney: Longman, 2nd edn, chap. 14, pp. 279–96.

Hearn, J. (1982) 'Notes on patriarchy, professionalisation and the semi-professions', *Sociology*, 16 (2), 184–202.

Helman, C.G. (1994) *Culture, Health, and Illness*, Oxford: Butterworth-Heinemann, 3rd edn.

Herzlich, C. (1973) *Health and Illness: A Social Psychological Analysis*, London: Academic Press.

Higgins, R., Hurst, K. and Wistow, G. (1999) *Psychiatric Nursing Revisited: The Care Provided for Acute Psychiatric Patients*, London: Whurr.

Horton, R. (1998) 'A stab in the back', *Observer*, 11 January.

Howarth, C., Kenway, P., Palmer, G. and Miorelli, R. (1999) *Monitoring Poverty and Social Exclusion*, London: The New Policy Institute/Joseph Rowntree Foundation.

Hughes, J. (1991) *An Outline of Modern Psychiatry*, Chichester: Wiley, 3rd edn.

Hugman, R. (1991) *Power in Caring Professions*, London: Macmillan.

Illich, I. (1977) 'Disabling Professions', in I. Illich, I. Zola, J. McKnight, J. Caplan and H. Shaiken (eds), *Disabling Professions*, Boston, MA: Marion Boyers, chap. 1, pp. 11–39.

Illsley, R. (1986) 'Occupational class, selection and the production of health inequalities in health', *Quarterly Journal of Social Affairs*, 2 (2), 151–65.

Joannides, P. and Gross, D. (1999) *The Guide to Getting it On!*, West Hollywood, CA: Goofy Foot Press

Jolley, M. (1989) 'The professionalisation of nursing: the uncertain path', in M. Jolley and P. Allan (eds), *Current Issues in Nursing*, London: Chapman and Hall.

Johnson, M. (1997) *Nursing and Social Judgement*, Aldershot: Ashgate.

Johnson, T. (1972) *Professions and Power*, London: Macmillan.

Johnstone, L. (1989) *Users and Abusers of Psychiatry: A Critical Look at Traditional Psychiatric Practice*, London: Routledge.

Jones, S. (ed.) (1995) *Cybersociety*, London: Sage.

Kinsey, A., Pomeroy, W. and Martin, C. (1948) *Sexual Behaviour in the Human Male*, Philadelphia, PA: Saunders.

—— (1953) *Sexual Behaviour in the Human Female*, Philadelphia, PA: Saunders.

Kramer, P.D. (1994) *Listening to Prozac: A Psychiatrist Explores Antidepressant Drugs and the Remaking of the Self*, London: Fourth Estate.

Kubler-Ross, E. (1969) *On Death and Dying*, New York: Macmillan.

Kuhn, T. (1962) *The Structure of Scientific Revolutions*, Chicago, IL: Chicago University Press.

Lacquer, T. (1990) *Making Sex: Body and Gender from the Greeks to Freud*, Cambridge, MA: Harvard University Press.

Layder, D. (1994) *Understanding Social Theory*, London: Sage.

Le Fanu, J. (1997) 'Rise of the non-disease', *Sunday Telegraph*, 7 December.

Lemert, E.M. (1951) *Social Pathology: A Systematic Approach to the Study of Sociopathic Behaviour*, New York: McGraw-Hill.

Lewis, A. (1953) 'Health as a social concept', *British Journal of Sociology*, 2 (4), 109–24.

Lorber, J. (1994) *Paradoxes of Gender*, New Haven, CT: Yale University Press.

Lukes, S. (1974) *Power: A Radical View*, London: Macmillan.

McIntosh, J. (1977) *Communication and Awareness in a Cancer Ward*, London: Croom Helm.

Macionis, J. and Plummer, K. (1998) *Sociology: A Global Perspective*, London: Prentice Hall, 3rd edn.

McKenna, H. (1999) *Nursing Theories and Models*, London: Routledge.

McKinlay, J. and Stoeckle, J. (1988) 'Corporization and the social transformation of doctoring', *International Journal of Health Services*, 18 (2), 191–205.

Maguire, K. and Campbell, D. (2000) 'Tobacco giant implicated in global smuggling schemes', *Guardian*, 31 January.

Marmot, M.G., Shipley, M.J. and Rose, G. (1984) 'Inequalities in death – specific explanations of a general pattern?', *Lancet*, i, 5 May, 1003–6.

Marmot, M.G., Smith, D. and Stansfeld, S.A. (1991) 'Health inequalities among British civil servants: the Whitehall Study II', *Lancet*, 337, 1387–93.

Marshall, T. (2000) 'Exploring fiscal food policy: the case of diet and ischaèmic heart disease', *British Medical Journal*, 320, 301–5.

Marx, K. (1844) *Economic and Philosophical Manuscripts of 1844*, ed. D. Struik and trans. M. Milligan, London: Lawrence and Wishart, 1959.

—— (1867) *Das Kapital/Capital: a Critique of Political Economy*, ed. F. Engels, London: Lawrence and Wishart, 1971.

Mathews, R. (1993) 'Squaring up to crime', *Sociological Review*, February, 26–9.

—— (1998) 'Flukes and flaws', *Prospect-Magazine*, 20–4 November.

Mechanic, D. (1968) *Medical Sociology*, New York: Free Press.

Medical Research Council (2000) *Call for Proposals: Human DNA Sample Collections from Patient Cohorts and Case/Control Studies*, London: Medical Research Council.

Meltzer, H., Baljit, G. and Petticrew, M. (1994) *Surveys of Psychiatric Morbidity among Adults aged 16–64 Living in Private Households in Great Britain*, London: Office of Population Census and Surveys.

Milburn, A. (1999) 'Health secretary spells out why beating disease can help win the wider war on inequality', *Guardian*, 12 December.

Millett, K. (1977) *Sexual Politics*, London: Virago.

Mills, C.W. (1959) *The Sociological Imagination*, Oxford: University of Oxford Press.

Morgan, M., Calnan, M. and Manning, N. (1985) *Sociological Approaches to Health and Medicine*, London: Croom Helm.

Morrall, P.A. (1998a) 'Clinical sociology and empowerment', in P. Barker and B. Davidson (eds), *Psychiatric Nursing: Ethical Strife*, London: Arnold.

—— (1998b) *Mental Health Nursing and Social Control*, London: Whurr.

—— (1999) 'Social exclusion and madness: the complicity of psychiatric medicine and nursing', in *Health and Social Exclusion*, London: Routledge, chap. 6, pp. 104–21.

—— (2000) *Madness & Murder*, London: Whurr.

Morrow, R. with Brown, D.D. (1994) *Critical Theory and Methodology*, London: Sage.

Mulkay, M. (1993) 'Social death in Britain', in D. Clark (ed.), *The Sociology of Death*, Oxford: Blackwell, chap. 2, pp. 31–49.

National Health Service Management Executive (1996) *Primary Care: The Future*, London: Department of Health.

National Institute for Clinical Excellence (1999) *What is the National Institute for Clinical Excellence?*, London: National Institute for Clinical Excellence.

Navarro, V. (1986) *Crisis, Health and Medicine: A Social Critique*, London: Tavistock.

Nie, N.H. and Erbring, L. (2000) *Internet and Society: A Preliminary Report*, Stanford, CA: Stanford Institute for the Quantitative Study of Society.

Nolan, P. (1993) *A History of Mental Health Nursing*, London: Chapman and Hall.

Nuland, S. (1996) 'An epidemic of discovery', *Time Magazine* (Special Issue), 148 (14), 8–13.

Office for National Statistics (1999) *Population Trends 98*, London: Stationery Office.

OPCS (1991) *Explanation of the Occupational Classification Scheme*, London: HMSO.

Oppenheimer, M. (1973) 'The proletarianisation of the professional', *Sociological Review Monograph*, 20, 213–37.

Parsons, T. (1951) *The Social System*, London: Routledge and Kegan Paul.

Popper, K. (1959) *The Logic of Scientific Discovery*, New York: Harper and Row.

Porter, R. (1987) *A Social History of Madness: Stories of the Insane*, London: Weidenfeld and Nicolson.

Porter, S. (1996) 'Contra-Foucault: soldiers, nurses and power', *Sociology*, 30 (1), 59–78.

Poulantzas, N. (1978) *State, Power, Socialism*, London: New Left Books.

Radford, T. (1999) 'Cracking the code of human life', *Guardian*, 2 December.

Radley, A. (1994) *Making Sense of Illness: The Social Psychology of Health and Disease*, London: Sage.

Rafferty, A.M. (1996) *The Politics of Nursing Knowledge*, London: Routledge.

Richman, J. (1987) *Medicine and Health*, London: Longman.

Robertson, A., Brunner, E. and Sheilam, A. (1999) 'Food is a political issue', in M. Marmot and R.G. Wilkinson (eds), *Social Determinants of Health*, Oxford: Oxford University Press, chap. 9, pp. 179–208.

Rose, D. and O'Reilly, K. (eds) (1997) *Constructing Classes: Towards a New Social Classification for the UK*, Swindon: ERSC/ONS.

Rose, S. (1997) *Lifelines: Biology, Freedom, Determinism*, Harmondsworth: Penguin.

Russell, B. (1961) *History of Western Civilisation*, London: Routledge.

Scase, R. (1999) *Britain towards 2010: The Changing Business Environment*, Swindon: Economic and Social Research Council.

Saks, M. (1995) *Professions and Public Interest*, London: Routledge.

Salvage, J. (1988) 'Professionalisation – or struggle for survival? A consideration of current proposals for the reform of nursing in the United Kingdom', *Journal of Advanced Nursing*, 13, 515–19.

Samson, C. (1995) 'The fracturing of medical dominance in British psychiatry', *Sociology of Health and Illness*, 17 (2), 245–69.

Sanger Centre (1999) *Information Release: Chromosome 22 Sequence Completed*, Cambridge: Sanger Centre.

Scambler, G. (1997) *Sociology as Applied to Medicine*, London: Saunders, 4th edn.

Scheerer, S. and Hess, H. (1997) 'Social control: a defence and reformulation', in R. Bergalli and C. Sumner (eds), *Social Control and Political Order: European Perspectives at the End of the Century*, chap. 5, pp. 96–130.

Scheff, T.J. (1966) *Being Mentally Ill: A Sociological Theory*, Chicago, IL: Aldine.

Scull, A.T. (1979) *Museums of Madness: The Social Organisation of Insanity in Nineteenth Century England*, Harmondsworth: Penguin.

—— (1984) *Decarceration: Community Treatment and the Deviant – A Radical View*, Cambridge: Polity Press, 2nd edn.

—— (1993) *The Most Solitary of Afflictions: Madness and Society in Britain, 1700–1900*, New Haven, CT: Yale University Press.

Seedhouse, D. (1991) *Liberating Medicine*, Chichester: Wiley.

Shorter, E. (1997) *A History of Psychiatry*, Wiley: New York.

Smail, D. (1984) *Illusion and Reality: The Meaning of Anxiety*, London: Dent.

Smith, P. (1993) 'Nursing as an occupation', in S. Taylor and D. Field (eds), *Sociology of Health and Health Care*, Oxford: Blackwell, chap. 12, pp. 205–33.

Sokal, A. and Bricmont, J. (1998) *Intellectual Impostures*, London: Profile Books.

Sontag, S. (1990) *Illness as Metaphor/AIDS and its Metaphors*, New York: Doubleday.

Stein, L. (1967) 'The doctor–nurse game', *Archives of General Psychiatry*, 12, 699–703.

Stone, M.H. (1998) *Healing the Mind: A History of Psychiatry from Antiquity to the Present*, London: Pimlico.

Sudnow, D. (1967) *Passing On: The Social Organisation of Dying*, New York: Prentice Hall.

Szasz, T.S. (1972) *The Myth of Mental Illness*, St Albans: Paladin.

—— (1973) *The Manufacture of Madness*, St Albans: Granada.

—— (1974) *The Myth of Mental Illness: Foundations for a Theory of Personal Conduct*, New York: Harper and Row.

—— (1993) 'Curing, coercing, and claims-making: a reply to critics', *British Journal of Psychiatry*, 162, 797–800.

—— (1994) 'Mental illness is still a myth', *Society*, 31 (4), 34–9.

—— (1998) 'Parity for mental illness, disparity for the mental patient', *Lancet*, 352 (9135), 1213–15.

Szasz, T. and Hollender, M.H. (1956) 'A contribution to the philosophy of medicine', *American Medical Association's Archives of Internal Medicine*, XCVII, 585–92.

Tannen, D. (1992) *You Just Don't Understand: Women and Men in Conversation*, London: Virago.

Timmermans, S. (1998) 'Social death as self-fulfilling prophecy: David Sudnow's *Passing On* revisited', *The Sociological Quarterly*, 39 (3), 453–72.

Townsend, P., Davidson, N. and Whitehead, M. (1992) *Inequalities in Health: The Black Report; The Health Divide*, Harmondsworth: Penguin, 2nd edn.

Townsend, P., Phillimore, P. and Beattie, A. (1987) *Health and Deprivation: Inequality in the North*, London: Croom Helm.

Travis, A. (1999) 'Sex in the 90s: the young take a moral stand', *Guardian*, 29 December.

Turner, B.S. (1995) *Medical Power and Social Knowledge*, London: Sage, 2nd edn.

UKCC (1999) *Practitioner–Client Relationships and the Prevention of Abuse*, London: UKCC.

United Nations/World Health Organisation (1998) *Report on the Global HIV/AIDS Epidemic*, New York: UN/WHO.

Vliet, Virginia van der (1996) *The Politics of Aids*, London: Bowerdean.

Wainwright, P. (1994) 'Professionalism and the concept of role extension', in G. Hunt and P. Wainwright (eds), *Expanding the Role of the Nurse: The Scope of Professional Practice*, Oxford: Blackwell, chap. 1, pp. 3–21.

Walker, M. (1998) 'Clinton and Blair set date for Third Way conference', *Guardian*, 14 August.

Walter, Tony (1991) 'Modern death: taboo or not taboo?', *Sociology*, 25 (2), 293–310.

Waters, M. (1994) *Modern Sociological Theory*, London: Sage.

Wazir, B. (1999) 'Life at the end of the line', *Observer*, 21 November.

Weber, M. (1948) *From Max Weber: Essays in Sociology*, trans. and ed. H.H. Gerth and C.W. Mills, London: Routledge and Kegan Paul.

West, P. (1991) 'Rethinking the health selection explanation for health inequalities', *Social Science and Medicine*, 32, 373–84.

White, M. (2000) 'Team of outsiders to drive NHS reform', *Guardian*, 24 February.

Whitehead, M. (1992) 'The health divide', in P. Townsend, N. Davidson and M. Whitehead (eds), *Inequalities in Health: The Black Report; The Health Divide*, Harmondsworth: Penguin, 2nd edn, pp. 219–438.

Wilkinson, A. (1997) 'Sorry state in the States', *Guardian*, 12 August.

Wilkinson, R.G. (1999) 'Putting the picture together: prosperity, redistribution, health, and welfare', in M. Marmot and R.G. Wilkinson (eds), *Social Determinants of Health*, Oxford: Oxford University Press, chap. 12, pp. 256–74.

Witz, A. (1992) *Profession and Patriarchy*, London: Routledge.

Woolf, M. and Illman, J. (1998) 'Food giants want you to eat more of this – even if it kills you', *Observer*, 7 June.

World Bank (1993) *World Development Report 1993*, New York: Oxford University Press.

World Health Organisation (1946) *Constitution of the World Health Organisation*, Geneva: WHO.

—— (1978) *Alma-Ata 1977 (Health for All) Declaration*, Copenhagen: WHO.

—— (1999) *World Health Report: Global Disease Burden – Leading Causes of Mortality and Burden of Disease, Estimates for 1998*, Geneva: World Health Organisation.

—— (2000) *World Health Report 2000*, Geneva: WHO.

Young, M. and Cullen, L. (1996) *A Good Death: Conversations with East Londoners*, London: Routledge.

Zola, I. (1977) 'Healthism and disabling medicalization', in I. Illich, I. Zola, J. McKnight, J. Caplan and H. Shaiken (eds), *Disabling Professions*, Boston, MA: Marion Boyers, chap. 2, pp. 41–67.

Index